NATURALLY

Bug-Free

75 Nontoxic Recipes

for Repelling Mosquitoes, Ticks, Fleas, Ants,
Moths & Other Pesky Insects

STEPHANIE L. TOURLES

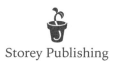

Storey Publishing

The mission of Storey Publishing is to serve our customers by publishing practical information that encourages personal independence in harmony with the environment.

Edited by Deborah Balmuth and Lisa Hiley
Art direction and book design by Jeff Stiefel
Indexed by Samantha Miller

Cover photograph by © Alexandra Grablewski
Illustrations by © Zoë More O'Ferrall/Illustrationweb.com

Read the instructions carefully and follow the safety precautions completely when making recipes. Consult a veterinarian before introducing any new treatment to your pet. This book is not intended to replace professional medical or veterinary advice or treatment.

Storey Publishing
210 MASS MoCA Way
North Adams, MA 01247
www.storey.com

Printed in the United States by Dickinson Press
10 9 8 7 6 5 4 3 2 1

Library of Congress Cataloging-in-Publication Data on file

Contents

Dedication

To anyone who's ever been stung, bitten, irritated, disgusted, annoyed, driven mad, or terrified by common insects and household pests — Mother Nature has the natural and safe solution.

May you be bugged, boggled, and pestered no more!

Acknowledgments

I give thanks to God above for the herbs and to the plant spirits themselves for imparting their knowledge; to my grandfather, Earl C. Ashe, for introducing me to folk herbalism as a young girl; to my friends and family for their feedback on my formulations; and to Deborah Balmuth, my chief editor at Storey Publishing, for believing in me once again and allowing me to share my herbal wisdom for the benefit of my health-seeking readers.

INTRODUCTION

We all hate those annoying pests that plague us on picnics, pounce on our pets, and parade through our pantries. We battle them inside and out: mosquitoes, fleas, ticks, biting flies, clothes and pantry moths, flour and grain beetles and mites, stinkbugs, ants, cockroaches, spiders, silverfish, earwigs, gnats, houseflies, fruit flies, centipedes, pill bugs, and so many other crawling, flying creatures.

I hear all the time from people looking for alternatives to the standard chemical arsenal that is available to repel or control insects and pests. I've made my own herb-based repellent products for years. They smell pleasant and work quite well, though I admit that when deerflies and blackflies (the latter are jokingly referred to where I live as the "Maine State Bird") are particularly voracious, I don protective clothing or stay indoors.

My cats, too, no longer suffer skin and respiratory irritation from flea-and-tick powders and those liquid "spot-on" products. I've perfected herbal formulations that keep them comfortable and healthy and, as a bonus, smelling fresh and clean. And I use herbs and other natural ingredients to keep my quaint country home, built in 1800, free of bugs and mice.

Many herbs emit powerfully aromatic volatile oils that, while appealing to most humans, repel many bugs and rodents, whose sense of smell is far more acute than ours. Certain herbs, such as tansy, wormwood, and pennyroyal, and other natural ingredients, such as pure borax and diatomaceous earth, act as insecticides rather than mere repellents; when used properly, however, they are harmless to people, animals, and the environment.

The Problem with Modern Insecticides

If you look at chemical insecticides purely from the standpoint of their intended benefit, they should be considered a scientific success, being tremendously effective against insects that transmit disease and damage crops and property. But that's where the success stops. Chemical insecticides, even when properly applied (not to mention when used carelessly or excessively), also kill beneficial insects, birds, and small mammals. Eventually many species of insects become resistant or immune. In addition, some insecticides, notably DDT, tend to persist in the environment, eventually accumulating in the body tissues of wildlife, fish, and humans.

Three of the most common, broad-spectrum insecticides used in the United States today are outlined below. All are neurotoxins that disrupt nerve impulses, then kill or disable insects in short order. Altogether, they are registered for use on over 100 different crops, animals, ornamental plants, and indoor areas.

THE ORGANOPHOSPHATES (OPs), which include chlorpyrifos, diazinon, malathion, and parathion, among others, are a family of household and agricultural insecticides. Many that have been in use for decades are at the top of the Environmental Protection Agency's hazardous chemical list. OPs are also used in military settings and by terrorists as chemical warfare nerve agents and have a cumulative effect, meaning that multiple exposures amplify the toxicity. Of all pesticides, these are the most toxic to vertebrates.

CARBAMATE INSECTICIDES, which include carbaryl (marketed as Sevin), are similar to organophosphates, but they break down more quickly. One EPA report describes them this way: "very broad spectrum toxicity and highly toxic to fish, bees, and parasitic wasps."

PYRETHROIDS, supposedly the least toxic and least persistent of the three types, are frequently used in household insecticides, on many food crops, on ornamental plants and lawns, and in veterinary products. Permethrin, a type of pyrethroid, is the most common active ingredient in indoor/outdoor insect sprays and has been classified by the EPA as "likely to be carcinogenic to humans." It is used in indoor fogging systems, and in city and suburban mosquito misting systems. Pyrethroids are extremely toxic to fish, as well as bees and other beneficial insects.

DEET: THE BEST DEFENSE?

Developed in the 1940s by the U.S. Army for protection of military personnel in insect-infested areas and registered in the U.S. for use by the general public in the mid-1950s, N-diethyl-m-toluamide (DEET) is one of the most widely used ingredients in store-bought, conventional bug sprays for personal use. It is a colorless, oily liquid with a mild odor and is designed to repel, rather than kill, insects, including mosquitoes, biting flies, fleas, ticks, and other small insects.

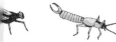

DEET is used by an estimated one-third of the U.S. population each year. Its use has increased dramatically since the 1970s as an aid to protect against Lyme disease, Rocky Mountain spotted fever, and other tick-borne illnesses, as well as West Nile virus. Although it clearly works as intended, it is not safe — even the EPA, as well as the product package label, says that you should wash it off your skin when you return indoors, avoid breathing it in, and not spray it directly on your face. A known eye irritant, it can cause rashes, soreness, or blistering.

A mosquito repellent containing 25 percent DEET cannot be applied on or near plastic, leather, synthetic fabrics, watch crystals, or painted or varnished surfaces, including automobiles. If this chemical, which in addition to being toxic to insects is also toxic to birds and aquatic life, can damage plastic, leather, and glass, then what is it doing to you? Remember that your skin is your largest organ, and it can absorb up to 60 percent of what you put on it!

SIDE EFFECTS OF INSECTICIDES

All chemical insecticides, whether applied in vapor, liquid, or powder form, have potentially toxic side effects if the vapors are inhaled, the product is orally consumed (for example, by a pet licking its fur), or through dermal exposure. Side effects can include nausea, headache, irritability, skin irritation, tremors, weakness, blurry vision, convulsions, vomiting, abdominal cramps, twitching, confusion, and/or difficulty breathing. Chronic exposure may lead to disorientation, speech difficulties, sleep disturbances, eye pain, and/or behavioral disorders. Each year, millions of people report suffering medically significant side effects from the use of insecticides.

When chemical-based insecticides are sprayed in the home, the vapors evaporate and can recondense on furniture, bedding, and objects such as toys. Young children, who spend a lot of time putting things in their mouths, are far more vulnerable than adults to such exposure.

As for pet products, some dogs and cats react badly to chemical-based flea and tick products (spot-on liquid insecticide or powder). Shortly after application, they might roll about on the ground, become hyperactive, flick their paws, twitch their skin or ears, or salivate excessively. After a few hours, they may exhibit lethargy and fatigue, indicate irritation of the mucous membranes and respiratory tract, and develop dermatitis. These products are supposed to be applied to your pet's skin, but the precautionary statement indicates that getting them on your own skin is not a good thing. What the heck? And those convenient pills that make your pet's blood poisonous to fleas and ticks don't seem any safer to me.

It's Time for a Change!

We have sprayed and sprinkled pesticides throughout our planet, which we share with all other life forms. Chemicals can be found in our blood, fatty tissue, and urine. They are present in our exhaled breath. As consumers, we don't have to add to the problem. We can take responsibility and remove as many poisons as we can from our homes and food chain. We can stop purchasing and using chemical-based products and do a "green housecleaning" to rid our homes of them (being careful to dispose of them properly, of course).

We can make safer products that won't make us or our pets sick or pollute our homes, let alone lead to insecticide resistance or immunity and permanently harm our beautiful Earth. I wrote this book to show people how easy it is to transition from synthetic repellents and pest controls to all-natural formulas. While herbal remedies for health and beauty are enjoying a renaissance, herb-based insecticides and repellents remain relatively unfamiliar, though I guarantee that our great-grandparents knew how to use them for that purpose.

These all-natural formulations are fun and simple to make! You have nothing to lose except the bugs that pester you and your pets, and a lot to gain — a more comfortable you; happier, healthier pets; and a fresh-smelling, bug-free home!

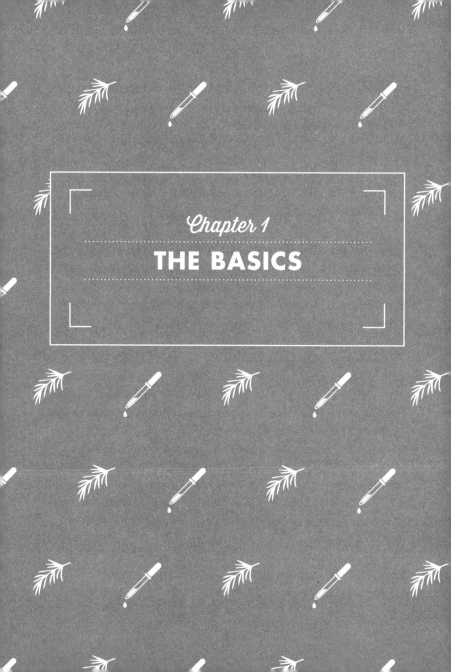

Chapter 1

THE BASICS

This chapter covers the four categories of ingredients that I use in my formulations and should help you understand how and why I constructed each recipe. If this is your first foray into crafting herbal repellents, or any herbal products, your head might be spinning — some of the ingredients may seem foreign to you. Fortunately, most of them are readily available at health food stores, food co-ops, and whole foods grocers. In season, a good farmers' market can be a wonderful source for fresh herbs.

The Internet, of course, is a go-to resource for just about everything you'll need. I grow many of my own herbs, but some, along with other necessary ingredients, I purchase from trusted mail-order catalogs or online sources. I prefer sources that have a relatively rapid turnover of stock, so that I can be sure the ingredients are fresh (see Resources, page 170).

If you have room for a garden, you too can grow many of these herbs. Most bug-repellent and insecticidal herbs are rather hardy and can withstand quite a bit of neglect. And if you are lucky enough to locate a local herb farm and apothecary, you'll think you've died and gone to do-it-yourself heaven. What a glorious resource for fresh and dried herbs, herb blends, beeswax, and base oils, plus many professionally made remedies (including, perhaps, a few nontoxic insect repellents) for you to sample. Herb farms often have public gardens to stroll through, and many offer classes in all manner of herb studies. A visit would be well worth your time!

An Ingredient Primer

If you know a little about herbal products for topical medicine or body care, then you are probably familiar with some of these ingredients. If you're a novice, no worries — here is an in-depth introduction to four categories of general ingredients: herbs, essential oils, base oils, and ethyl alcohol. Before you purchase any ingredients and start stirring and straining, pouring and packaging, take a few minutes to educate yourself. A knowledge-able consumer makes the wisest choices and the highest-quality handmade preparations.

Herbs

I suggest you look the various herbs up in a few different herb books; study their uses, both historical and current; and learn their growth habits, harvesting and storage requirements, and any contraindications. Learning about herbs can be quite fascinating! But don't stop there: try to grow the plants or ethically wild-harvest them, if you can, and get to know them on their own turf, where they're energetic, green, and alive. At the very least, become familiar with various herbs in their dried state.

The herbs called for in this book are relatively common, easy to find, and used in dried form unless otherwise specified. If you have access to freshly grown herbs, then you may want to dry and process them yourself, using the following instructions. Recently processed herbs smell wonderful, and their components are at their peak — they'll make your products all the more delightful and effective.

HARVESTING HERBS

You may be surprised by how easy it is to dry and process fresh herbs. With any technique, it's best to dry the herbs as soon as they're picked (or purchased) to fully preserve their beneficial properties. Here are some key points.

- Always use a sharp knife or hand pruners to cut herbs.

- Gather herbs in early to mid-morning, just after any dew has dried but before it's too hot.

- Harvest flowers or flowering tops, such as yarrow, when the flowers have just opened. Harvest buds, such as lavender, when the buds are mature and well formed, but have not yet opened.

- Chose herbs that are free of insects and disease and have not been treated with pesticides.

- Handle herbs carefully to avoid bruising.

- Herbs should be relatively dirt-free, but if they're dusty, rinse them quickly in cool water and immediately pat them dry with a paper towel or soft, lint-free cloth or give them a quick spin in salad spinner. To remove dirt from harvested roots, gently scrub with a vegetable brush and then rinse them thoroughly. (Many herbalists who grow their own herbs or harvest from wild, clean places don't rinse their herbs prior to use. I do recommend rinsing all purchased fresh herbs.)

DRYING HERBS

Herbs can take from four days to several weeks to dry completely, depending on weather conditions and the thickness of the material. Roots, bark, twigs, seeds, nut hulls, and rinds take the longest. The ideal temperature for drying is between 65 and 85°F (18°–30°C). When herbs are ready, leaves and stems are brittle, but not dry enough to shatter; flower petals and buds feel semi-crisp; roots and rinds are hard or ever-so-slightly pliable; and barks, twigs, seeds, and nut hulls are very hard and dry.

Avoid overdrying herbs; it can diminish their valuable properties. No matter what part of the plant you are drying, never let it go to the point that it crumbles into dust when squeezed. Store dried herbs in airtight containers in a cool, moisture-free place away from direct sunlight, for up to one year.

Hang-Drying Herbs

To dry herbs by hanging them, gather a small handful of stems of a single variety into a bundle fastened with string or a rubber band. Many herbs look similar when dried, so I recommend labels. Hang the bundles upside down in a well-ventilated, dimly lit area with low humidity. Leave plenty of room between bundles to ensure good air circulation and to keep scents from mingling.

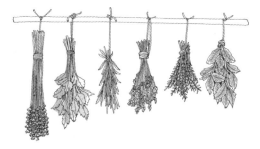

Screen-Drying Herbs

Most herbs can be successfully dried on screens, either repurposed window screens or ones made specifically for drying herbs and foods. I prefer screens made with nylon mesh, but wire mesh works fine. Just be sure to clean them thoroughly and remove any rust before using them.

To prepare herbs, spread them in a single layer by type — for example, flowers, leaves, roots, or bark — leaving space for good air circulation. Place the screens in a well-ventilated, dimly lit area with low humidity. I set mine atop small blocks of wood in my garden shed. Stacking the screens is fine, as long as you allow for adequate ventilation.

If you're setting up screens outside on a dry, sunny day, put them in a mostly shady area protected from wind. Cover the plant material with a single layer of cheesecloth, if you wish, to keep out airborne debris. Keep an eye on the weather and bring the screens in at night to avoid the evening dew.

Using a Food Dehydrator

A food dehydrator works quite well for processing herbs. Follow the manufacturer's instructions for placement of the herbs in the machine, but don't set the temperature any higher than 110°F (44°C) to preserve the color, fragrance, volatile oils, and chemical integrity.

EASY-TO-GROW "BUG OFF" PLANTS

Myriad herbs can be grown in pots, flowerbeds, or near lawns or vegetable gardens, where they emit chemicals into the air and/or soil that repel bugs and small rodents. Many are happy in most soil types and require little maintenance (unless potted), providing there is good drainage and the soil has been well prepared. Here are some my favorite herbs that offer protection where they grow and can be dried for future uses. In many cases, the freshly harvested leaves and stems can be rubbed directly onto people and pets for instant relief from pests.

Anise	**Pennyroyal**
Basil	**Pyrethrum**
Bay laurel, tree	**Rosemary**
Bayberry, shrub	**Sage, culinary**
Calendula	**Sage, white**
Catnip	**Southernwood**
Chives	**Sweet woodruff**
Chrysanthemum	**Tansy**
Feverfew	**Thyme, culinary**
Garlic	**Thyme, lemon**
Geranium	**Tobacco, ornamental**
Hyssop	**Wormwood**
Lavender	**Yarrow**
Marigold	
Mint	
Mugwort	
Onion	

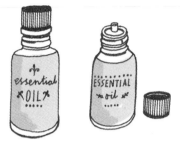

Essential Oils

Essential oils are often called the "life force" or "soul" of the plant, embodying its aromatic phytohormones and many powerful compounds. With regard to the crafting of bug-repelling and insecticide products, essential oils provide concentrated, fragrant, natural solutions to myriad pest problems.

Depending on the plant, essential oils are stored in either tiny cellular reservoirs or intercellular spaces and are even used by the plants themselves as repellents against damaging pests. Pure essential oils are extracted from various plant parts — grass, leaves, flowers, bark, rind, needles, berries, wood, roots, seeds, or resin — primarily by steam distillation, with the exception of citrus oils, which are generally cold-pressed from the fruit's rind.

Solvent extraction, another method used to extract essential oils from plants, uses petroleum-derived solvents, such as petroleum ether, hexane, toluene, butane, methane, and propane. The resultant oils are called *absolutes* and should be used for natural perfumery blending only, not aromatherapeutic use, as solvent residues may be present.

A newer method of extraction is supercritical carbon dioxide (CO_2) extraction, a more expensive yet superior process conducted under high pressure and relatively low heat without the use of steam or added solvents. This process results in superior fragrance quality and physiological activity.

Chemically, essential oils have nothing in common with base oils (see page 23). They do not contain fatty acids, are not prone to rancidity, and, because of their minute molecular makeup, they evaporate easily (hence their other common name, volatile oils). Essential oils blend quite readily with base oils and other fats, and they dissolve in 95 percent ethyl alcohol, and to some degree in 80- and 100-proof ethyl alcohol, making them an ideal formulary ingredient. They react with water much as fatty oils do — by floating to the top — but they readily lend their scent to water and other liquids, such as aloe vera gel, witch hazel, and vinegar.

BUYING AND USING ESSENTIAL OILS

As typical of all plant extracts, the concentration of active ingredients varies from batch to batch. The variation depends upon factors such as the geography, growing methods, soil fertility, and seasonal fluctuations, plus the age of the plant at harvest, and processing and extraction procedures. Thus, the effectiveness of the essential oils to repel or kill bugs can vary greatly. It pays to buy the highest-quality essential oils you can afford, preferably organic or wild-harvested — a little goes a long, long way.

Essential oils are usually liquid, but some are quite viscous (vetiver and patchouli, for example) or even semisolid (such as peppermint), depending on the temperature. To measure a thicker essential oil, set the bottle in a shallow bowl of warm water until it liquifies or warm the bottle between your palms for a few minutes (this doesn't work with cold hands!).

If you are serious about purchasing and using real, quality essential oils, I suggest that you read a couple of good books on the subject and take an aromatherapy class, if possible. I also recommend that you call the company whose oils you want to use and talk to a representative about the origins of their oils and their production methods. I purchase my essential oils from a handful of companies I've come to know and trust (see Resources, page 170).

Storing Essential Oils

Essential oils retain their healing properties for 5 to 10 years if properly stored in a dark, dry, cool place. The exception to this is citrus oils: They will remain potent for only 6 to 12 months unless refrigerated. When refrigerated, they may last for a couple of years if not opened frequently.

To prolong the shelf life of an essential oil, do not store it in a bottle with a rubber dropper top. The strong vapors will gradually weaken the rubber and allow air to enter the bottle, and the precious volatile beneficial properties will evaporate prematurely. Always purchase essential oils in bottles with a plastic-lined screw-on cap and use a sterile glass eyedropper to extract what you need; or make sure the bottle is sealed with a built-in drop-by-drop reducer cap, which is how most essential oil bottles under 2 ounces are sold.

Store Herbal Products Away from Children and Pets

Store all your herbal supplies and handcrafted products safely away from children and pets. All ingredients, essential oils in particular, have the potential to be toxic if ingested or applied to the skin improperly. Be especially mindful of culinary citrus oils, as they look and smell like fruity candy — store them on the top shelves of your kitchen cabinets away from eyesight and easy reach.

Essential oils are safe for use on children if used as directed in a particular child-safe recipe, but if swallowed, inhaled excessively, poured on the skin, or rubbed into the eyes or mucous membranes, they could be extremely irritating and debilitating, if not fatal.

ESSENTIAL OIL SAFETY TIPS

Essential oils are highly concentrated forms of herbal chemical energy, and they must be used with caution. Very few essential oils may be used neat (undiluted) on the skin, the exceptions being oils such as lavender, tea tree, patchouli, and rose geranium (and only 1 to 3 drops per day if used in this manner). Always dilute an essential oil in a base oil unless you know it's safe to use neat. It's important to educate yourself about the properties of and contraindications for each essential oil before you use it.

If you rub or splash an essential oil into your nose or eyes — which can cause excruciating pain — immediately flush the affected area with an unscented, bland fatty oil such as olive, almond, corn, soybean, peanut, or generic vegetable oil— whatever you have on hand. Full-fat cream, half-and-half, or whole milk makes an acceptable substitute in an emergency. Using plain water does not help; essential oils are attracted to fats alone. Should the pain continue or should severe headache or respiratory irritation develop, seek prompt medical attention and take the essential oil bottle with you. Most medical staff are unfamiliar with essential oils, so knowing exactly what they are dealing with will help in your treatment.

How to Do an Essential Oil Patch Test

Combine a drop or two of the essential oil in question with ½ teaspoon base oil, such as almond, soybean, jojoba, or coconut, in a tiny bowl. Soak a cotton ball with the liquid and tape it to the inside of your elbow or wrist; leave it for 12 to 24 hours. If the area becomes sore, itchy, or red, do not use this ingredient in your personal bug-repelling recipes.

Base Oils

Derived from beans, nuts, seeds, flowers, fruits, and grains, base oils are chemically classified as fats — they contain fatty acids and glycerin. Many are vegetable oils used in cooking, and you may also hear them called *unctuous oils*, *fixed oils*, or *carrier oils*. Base oils are characteristically greasy, slippery, smooth in texture, and lighter than water, with an extremely low evaporation rate. As their name implies, these oils are used as a base or carrying agent to which essential oils, solid fats, herbs, or spices are added.

I use only plant-derived fats, never lanolin, lard, cod liver oil, or mineral oil. In addition to being animal products, which I prefer to avoid, the first three are thick, don't penetrate the skin well, and often smell bad in formulations. Mineral oil can clog pores and is a petroleum by-product, which most people want to avoid.

When warmed, base oils extract and absorb herbal components such as essential oils, gums, resins, and oleoresins. Flavonoids, alkaloids, and other active principles are partially soluble in warm oil. A wonderful benefit derived from using base oils in insect-repelling formulations is that they evaporate slowly, leaving a skin-conditioning barrier on the skin's surface while delivering protection that lasts a bit longer than that provided by repellents based in water, witch hazel, or alcohol.

The best base oils are organically grown, naturally extracted, and minimally processed. The key words to look for on the label are *organic*, *cold-pressed* or *expeller-pressed*, or *unrefined* — these guarantee the highest quality. These oils have not been exposed to extraction procedures using petroleum-derived solvents, such as hexane, nor to extremely high temperatures, deodorizing, or bleaching. These processes can destroy or alter an oil's natural molecular state, affecting aroma, color, flavor, and consistency, as well as its antioxidant properties and vitamin, mineral, and essential fatty acid content.

It's important to note that most unrefined base oils — with the exception of coconut, extra-virgin olive, jojoba, and sesame — have a relatively short shelf life and tend to become rancid if stored at room temperature for more than eight months, especially in warm weather. These oils should be refrigerated and used within one year.

Purchase your oils through reputable retailers with a high turnover of inventory, and always check the expiration date on the bottle.

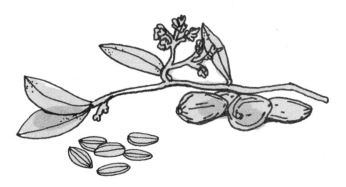

Ethyl Alcohol

Ethyl alcohol is used by herbalists as a menstruum (solvent) for extracting an herb's chemical components. Ninety-five percent ethyl alcohol (190 proof), also known as pharmaceutical grade alcohol, is sold in some states under the brand names Everclear and Clear Spring. Made from grains, it dissolves and extracts the alcohol-soluble constituents in plants — resins, fats, essential oils, fixed oils, alkaloids, coloring pigments, acrid and bitter compounds, alkaloidal salts, glycosides, organic acids, chlorophyll, uncrystallized sugars, and waxes.

There is more water in 80- or 100-proof ethyl alcohol, so it additionally extracts water-soluble constituents such as mucilage, gums, crystallized sugars, polysaccharides, saponins, tannins, and proteins. Ethyl alcohol is an excellent preservative. Alcohol-based herbal extracts last many years, while purely water-based "herbal tea" solutions degrade in a matter of days.

To make an alcoholic extract, the dried or fresh herb is chopped, mashed, or powdered, then macerated (soaked) in the alcohol for 2 to 8 weeks. Tougher materials such as bark, roots, and seeds require a longer soaking than more tender plant parts such as flowers and leaves. After soaking, the plant material is strained and squeezed out, leaving a tincture or herbal alcohol. Any chemicals that cannot be extracted into an alcohol-based solution remain in the marc (the strained plant residue).

As an insect-repellent spray base for humans, a tincture is convenient to apply, readily delivers its insect-repelling properties, and is generally pleasant to use, as it has a cooling effect on the skin as the alcohol evaporates. An herbal tincture can also be used as a base when making insecticidal sprays for the home.

I typically use 80-proof ethyl alcohol (which is 40 percent alcohol and 60 percent water). Ethyl alcohol is commonly called grain alcohol because it used to be made primarily from fermented corn. It is also made by fermenting rye, wheat, potatoes, molasses, or fruit, in which case it's known as whiskey, vodka, rum, brandy, or gin. I always use a very inexpensive brand of vodka, with no added sweeteners or flavoring; there's no need to waste money on premium brands.

Caution: Do not use isopropyl alcohol, as it is highly toxic if ingested and can be quite irritating to the skin.

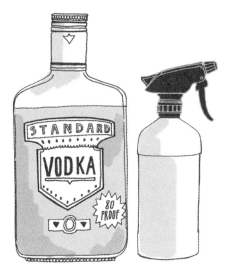

NATURAL ITCH AND STING RELIEF

Insects may be small, but their bites and stings can deliver a big dose of itchy, inflamed misery! Fortunately, many natural remedies work amazingly well to counteract this discomfort.

ALOE VERA JUICE OR GEL soothes the skin and relieves inflammation and itchiness. The juice is available commercially; just apply it directly on the skin with a cotton ball (it feels especially nice chilled) or dab the gel from a freshly cut leaf onto bites and stings.

APPLE CIDER VINEGAR is acidic, so it helps neutralize the alkaline venom injected by wasps, yellow jackets, and hornets. Apply a soaked cotton ball directly to stings for 30 minutes, refreshing the vinegar repeatedly.

BAKING SODA, in contrast to vinegar and lemon juice, is alkaline, so it helps neutralize the acidic venom of bees, ants, and other biting/stinging insects (other than wasps, yellow jackets, and hornets). Apply a paste of baking soda and water directly to irritated, inflamed areas and leave on for at least 30 minutes. Rinse. For an overall anti-itch remedy, add 1 cup of baking soda to a tub of lukewarm water and soak for 15 to 20 minutes.

continued

CLAY (BENTONITE, FRENCH GREEN, RED, OR WHITE) is one of the most overlooked, inexpensive healing substances around. Composed of myriad mineral deposits, it has remarkable absorbing and drawing powers; when thickly applied and allowed to dry, it actually raises the skin's temperature, increasing circulation and encouraging the release of toxins. To use, form a paste of powdered clay and a small amount of water, aloe vera juice, or peppermint tea. Apply it directly to the bite, and leave on for at least 30 minutes. Rinse.

LAVENDER OR TEA TREE ESSENTIAL OIL can be applied "neat," or undiluted, by the drop, directly to each bite to reduce inflammation and help prevent infection (1 to 3 drops of either oil maximum per day). These energetically cooling, concentrated oils are gentle, inexpensive, and very effective medicine! No natural first-aid kit should be without either one of them.

LEMON JUICE can be used just like apple cider vinegar.

NEEM OIL is a naturally cooling oil with antibacterial properties. It relieves many types of skin irritations. Apply a drop to each bite.

PLANTAIN — yes, the common "weed" — is cooling and has astringent, vulnerary (tissue healing), and anti-inflammatory properties, plus the leaves contain a wonderful mucilaginous substance that is quite soothing to skin irritations of all kinds. To use it fresh, find a clean, medium-size leaf, free from pesticide, roadside, or animal contamination, chew it to a pulp, and apply the "spit paste" to the affliction.

To use dried plantain, mix the chopped herb with a small amount of water and apply to the bite or sting. Either way you use it, within minutes of application, the area will become warm as toxins are drawn from the skin. Reapply as often as needed until the pain and swelling has subsided. Drying your own is easy, or it can be ordered online.

....

TOBACCO "SPIT PASTE" is an age-old remedy — it works like a charm to counteract the pain of insect bites and stings, but if you don't want to chew tobacco (and I don't blame you), mix enough water or peppermint tea into 2 teaspoons of shredded pipe or cigarette tobacco to make a paste and apply it directly to the bite. Leave it on for at least 30 minutes or until the swelling is gone. **Note:** If irritation or redness occurs, remove the tobacco.

....

VICKS VAPORUB has well-known cooling and soothing properties. This longtime favorite salve can take the itch out of insect bites and calm inflammation. It also makes a wonderful repellent, due to the camphor, eucalyptus, menthol, cedar leaf, and thyme contained within the familiar little blue jar. Be aware that it uses petrolatum as the thick carrier base, in case you are sensitive to it or want to avoid petroleum products. Petroleum-tree rubs are available in better health food stores and may be worth a try.

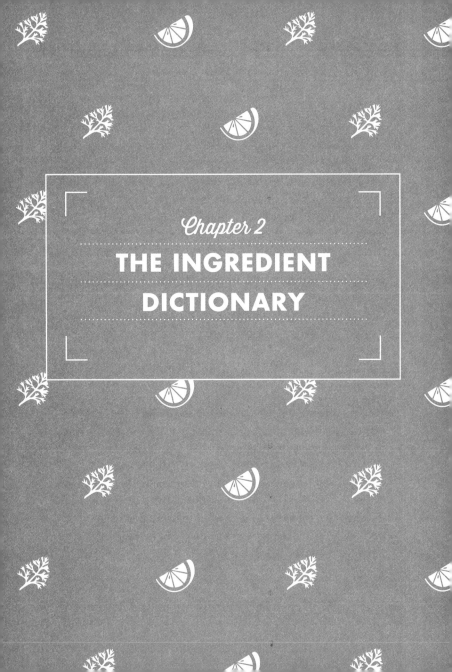

Chapter 2

THE INGREDIENT
DICTIONARY

This comprehensive listing of ingredients takes you on a descriptive journey through all the herbs and other natural ingredients called for in this book. Use it as a reference guide as you concoct your formulations, a process that is both educational and entertaining. Once you learn the basics of crafting homemade solutions to all things that "bug" you, you can develop your own formulations that please your senses and work best for your individual or family's and pet's needs.

Herbs and Botanical Ingredients

ANISE, STAR (*Illicium verum*)

The essential oil, derived from the licorice-scented seeds of this Oriental evergreen tree, has been used for centuries to fend off pesky outdoor insects. Its strong chemical components repel most bugs, especially mosquitoes, gnats, biting flies, moths, and houseflies. The whole or powdered seed pods can be added to insect-repellent sachets and placed in cupboards, clothes closets, armoires, and drawers.

PARTS USED: Essential oil, seeds

CAUTION: Avoid use of the essential oil if pregnant or epileptic.

BASIL, SWEET (*Ocimum basilicum*)

A member of the mint family, basil is a rather pungent culinary herb that is a mild to moderately effective insecticide and repellent against mosquitoes and their larvae, as well as chiggers, gnats, fleas, ticks, and houseflies. The fresh leaves are often used when making insect repellent sprays for people and pets, and the dried leaves can be used in sachets, or made into a tea and used as a final rinse after shampooing your pet.

PART USED: Leaves

SUBSTITUTE: Fresh lemon basil (*Ocimum basilicum citriodorum*) leaves can be rubbed onto the skin to help repel all manner of biting bugs, and also dried and used in household bug-repellent sachets.

BAY LAUREL (*Laurus nobilis*)

The bay leaf is a familiar culinary spice and also a terrific household bug repellent, especially for clothing and pantry moths, and flour and grain beetles and mites. Placing several leaves in stored whole grain and flour repels hungry grain pests. Keep a sachet of crushed bay leaves mixed with other strongly scented herbs such as black peppercorns, peppermint, wormwood, and patchouli, in cupboards, clothes closets, armoires, and drawers to help keep all manner of bugs at "bay" (pun intended!).

PART USED: Leaves

BLACK PEPPER (*Piper nigrum*)

This everyday kitchen spice, with its rather hot bite, repels a myriad of damaging insects such as clothing and pantry moths, flour and grain beetles and mites, spiders, silverfish, stinkbugs, ants, and cockroaches. I use it in insect-deterring potpourri bags and insecticidal powder blends.

PART USED: Peppercorns — whole and ground

CAMPHOR, WHITE (*Cinnamomum camphora*)

Derived from the leaves and bark of a tall evergreen tree that is native to China, Japan, Vietnam, and Taiwan, camphor essential oil has a rather strong woodsy/menthol/cardamom aroma. It is an effective moth repellent that works just as well as toxic, harsh-smelling mothballs. Always use "white" camphor. The "yellow," "blue," and "brown" versions are derived from the same tree but produced from heavier fractions of the oil; they contain large quantities of the chemical constituent safrole, a known carcinogen that is highly toxic.

PART USED: Essential oil

CAUTIONS: Avoid use if pregnant or epileptic. Potential skin irritant.

CATNIP *(Nepeta cataria)*
ALSO KNOWN AS CATMINT OR CATSWORT

This member of the mint family, with its pungent earthy-minty scent, is well known for attracting cats, but the primary aromatic component, nepetalactone, also makes it a powerful yet safe repellent of mice, rats, mosquitoes, cockroaches, and myriad household insects. In a 2001 Iowa State University study, nepetalactone was demonstrated to be 10 times more effective at repelling mosquitoes than DEET. Catnip essential oil is effective in concentrations as low as 1 percent.

I sprinkle dried catnip in carpeted areas where my cats sleep and lounge. They munch on it, frolic in it, have fewer fleas, and smell good. It can also be made into a tea and used as a final rinse after shampooing your pet. The fresh, crushed leaves can be rubbed directly onto the fur of both cats and dogs as a mild insect repellent. White fur may be stained temporarily green, but it will quickly wear off. Some cats react strongly to catnip, so start with small amounts and gauge your own pet's reaction before doing this.

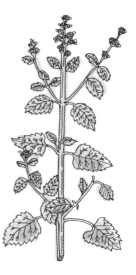

PARTS USED: Leaves and flowers, essential oil

CAUTION: Avoid use of the essential oil if pregnant or epileptic.

~~~~~~~~~~~~~~~

CAYENNE *(Capsicum annuum)*
The bright orange and red hot pepper flakes are used as an ingredient when

making insect-repelling potpourri bags. I use the dissolved powder in home insecticidal spray blends. Cayenne deters all manner of crawling insects from taking up residence in your home but works especially well against ants, cockroaches, spiders, silverfish, stinkbugs, and flour and grain beetles and mites.

PARTS USED: Pepper flakes and powder

SUBSTITUTE: A plain hot sauce such as Tabasco can be substituted for the powder in spray blends.

CAUTION: The volatile oils are extremely irritating to the eyes and mucous membranes. Wash hands immediately after working with cayenne.

~~~~~~~~~~~~~~~~~~~~~~~~~~~~~~~~~~~~~~~

CEDARWOOD, VIRGINIA *(Juniperus virginiana)*

This particular cedarwood is actually a type of juniper, not a member of the *Cedrus* genus. It is the source of most "cedar oil" on the market, as well as most wooden pencils. The essential oil as well as the fragrant, red-streaked wood (sold in plank, ball, block, and chip form) has been used for eons as a wonderful moth repellent.

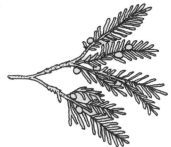

PARTS USED: Essential oil, wood

SUBSTITUTE: Texas cedarwood *(Juniperus mexicana)* essential oil and wood

CAUTION: Avoid use of the essential oil during pregnancy.

CINNAMON

(Cinnamomum zeylanicum, also known as *C. verum)*

The familiar hot, spicy, stimulating, sweet fragrance is derived from the bark of this tropical evergreen tree. This culinary herb has moderate insect-repelling properties, but I primarily use both the bark and essential oil to add a lovely aroma to herbal sachets that are to be placed in closets, drawers, and cabinets.

PARTS USED: Bark, essential oil

CAUTIONS: Avoid use of the essential oil if pregnant or epileptic. Severe skin irritant; must always be heavily diluted.

CITRONELLA *(Cymbopogon nardus)* OR JAVA CITRONELLA *(C. winterianus)*

A close relative of lemongrass, this familiar natural bug-repellent ingredient effectively repels mosquitoes, gnats, ants, moths, and other household bugs, so I use it in several of my formulations. If you find the earthy, slightly lemony aroma to be too heavy and cloying and prefer repellents that do not contain it, there are several effective substitutes.

PART USED: Essential oil

SUBSTITUTE: Essential oils of lemongrass, geranium, or lemon eucalyptus (eucalyptus citriodora, *Corymbia citriodora)*

CAUTIONS: Avoid if pregnant. May irritate very sensitive skin.

CLOVE *(Syzygium aromaticum; Eugenia caryophyllata)*

Cloves are actually the dried flower buds of a slender ever-green tree that is cultivated in tropical regions worldwide, but primarily Madagascar, the Philippines, and Indonesia. One of the oldest spices, it is super rich in the chemical constituent eugenol, which has amazing bug-repelling properties, especially effective against houseflies, gnats, mosquitoes, and clothing and pantry moths. I use both the essential oil and whole cloves in potpourri blends and occasionally use the essential oil in spray formulations for people.

PARTS USED: Whole cloves, essential oil

CAUTIONS: Avoid use of the essential oil if pregnant or epileptic. Severe skin irritant; must always be heavily diluted.

~~~~~~

EUCALYPTUS *(Eucalyptus globulus; E. radiata; E. smithii)*
There are over 700 different species of eucalyptus, of which at least 500 produce a type of essential oil. Eucalyptus essential oil has a familiar, strongly medicinal aroma with powerful insecticidal and repellent properties resulting from the volatile compound 1, 8 cineole, also known as eucalyptol (among others). When properly diluted, it is capable of killing numerous soft-bodied insects upon contact or will at least effectively repel them. Additionally, the dried aromatic leaves (typically *E. globulus*) and essential oil can be added to insect-repellent sachets and potpourri to repel mosquitoes, gnats, houseflies, cockroaches, silverfish, fleas, and ticks. Humans like the smell, but bugs do not!

E. globulus (blue gum eucalyptus) is the most pungent, sharp, camphorous, and penetrating of the three, and the only one with a cautionary warning (see below). *E. radiata* (grey eucalyptus or narrow-leaved peppermint eucalyptus) is preferred for its milder aroma and gentle nature upon the skin.

E. smithii (gully gum eucalyptus) has a dry, light odor and is gentle to the skin as well.

PARTS USED: Essential oil, leaves

SUBSTITUTE: Lemon eucalyptus (eucalyptus citriodora, *Corymbia citriodora*)

CAUTION: Avoid use of *E. globulus* essential oil if pregnant or epileptic.

Note: *E. radiata* and *E. smithii* are the gentlest of all eucalyptus species and are safe for pregnant and lactating women and for children and seniors.

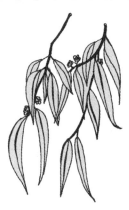

EUCALYPTUS, LEMON

(Eucalyptus citriodora; Corymbia citriodora)

This tall evergreen tree, native to Australia but cultivated primarily in China and Brazil, is also called lemon-scented eucalyptus. Derived from the leaves and twigs, this essential oil has a heavy, lemony-earthy, citronella-like aroma with strong insecticidal and repellent properties resulting from the primary volatile compound citronellal (among others) contained within. It can be used in the same manner as *Eucalyptus globulus*, listed above, and is especially effective against cockroaches and silverfish.

PART USED: Essential oil

SUBSTITUTE: *E. globulus, E. radiata,* or *E. smithii* essential oil

CAUTION: Avoid using *E. globulus* if pregnant or epileptic.

FEVERFEW *(Tanacetum parthenium)*

Feverfew shares the same genus with tansy and is grouped with the chrysanthemums and pyrethrums. With its extremely bitter flavor, combined with active chemical constituents such as sesquiterpene lactones, camphor, and pyrethrins, which act as potent pesticides and insect repellents, feverfew is a great addition to your natural bugs-be-gone arsenal. In fact, most household (and garden) bugs abhor its flavor and fragrance. The leaves and flowers can be utilized in many ways: crushed or ground in bug-repellent sachets or powders; made into a tincture and used as a mosquito-repellent base; or made into a tea and sprayed directly onto areas where bugs are a problem.

PARTS USED: Leaves and flowers

SUBSTITUTE: Tansy leaves and flowers

CAUTION: The fresh plant can irritate skin, so always wear gloves when harvesting.

GERANIUM *(Pelargonium graveolens)*

Distilled from the leaves of the rose geranium, a scented variety only distantly related to the common ornamental, this oil, with its pleasing rosy-citrus-green aroma, is an incredibly safe and gentle, highly effective mosquito and tick repellent for both humans and pets due to the chemical compounds citronellol and geraniol. Geraniol is often isolated to make synthetic rose oil and to extend real rose essential oil, as well as being added to commercially produced natural insect repellents. I use it quite often, especially during tick season, when I apply it by the drop to my clothing. Ticks hate it!

PART USED: Essential oil

LAVENDER (*Lavandula angustifolia*)

This familiar, popular herb, with the classic old-fashioned, sweet, floral fragrance, deters many insects, but traditionally, the dried flower buds and leaves were used in sachets to deter moths from destroying clothes, blankets, and other natural-fiber fabrics, especially those of animal origin. I use the essential oil, derived from the buds, in insect-repellent formulations, to inoculate fabric clothes hangers, in pet shampoos and pet bedding sachets, and in insect-deterrent formulations used to clean kitchen and bathroom cabinets.

PARTS USED: Flower buds and leaves, essential oil

LEMON (*Citrus × limon*)

With their sharp, uplifting aroma, lemons have been used for centuries to freshen the home and deter bugs. Limonene, a chemical extracted from citrus fruit peels, is often an active ingredient in many commercial home pesticide products, insect repellents, and flea- and tick-control products for dogs and cats. A few drops of lemon essential oil can be added to the washing machine when laundering pet bedding, as it acts as an insecticide for fleas, their eggs and larvae, and ticks, and it lends a fresh, clean scent. I also use the essential oil in insect-deterrent formulations used to clean kitchen and bathroom cabinets. Dried lemon peel and essential oil can be added to pet bedding sachets and household bug-repellent potpourris.

PARTS USED: Peel, essential oil

SUBSTITUTE: Sweet orange essential oil and peel; grapefruit essential oil and peel

CAUTIONS: Avoid use of the essential oil if pregnant or epileptic. May be photosensitizing and a potential skin irritant.

LEMONGRASS *(Cymbopogon citratus)*

Derived from the grasslike leaves, lemongrass essential oil has a pungent, lemony scent with an earthy undertone; the dried grass is much milder. Lemongrass essential oil deters mosquitoes, flour and grain beetles and mites, clothes and pantry moths, cockroaches, silverfish, fleas, and ticks. A cousin of citronella, it is incorporated in many commercial repellent sprays, and I use it often. The dried herb can be added to bug-repellent sachets.

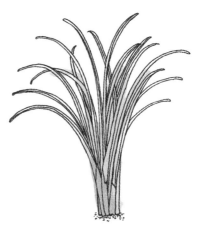

PARTS USED: Leaves, essential oil

CAUTIONS: Avoid use of the essential oil if pregnant or epileptic. May be photosensitizing and a possible skin irritant.

MUGWORT (*Artemisia annua; A. vulgaris*)

Though not quite as chemically strong, this silvery-leafed, sweetly pungent relative of wormwood — also known as sweet wormwood — has very bitter leaves that have been used for centuries in sachet blends as an effective moth repellent in kitchen cupboards, clothes closets, armoires, and drawers. Like wormwood, the leaves contain thujone and camphor, which are highly toxic to insect pests in the home and garden. I use the powdered leaves in flea repellent and insecticide blends for pets and carpeting.

PART USED: Leaves

SUBSTITUTE: Wormwood leaves

NEEM (*Azadirachta indica*)

The rich, thick, golden-brown base oil, with its rather strong nutty-earthy aroma, derived from pressed neem tree nuts, has wonderful insecticidal, antifungal, and repellent properties and is a commonly used ingredient in natural, commercial pesticide products. Typically, it's diluted with 15 to 20 percent olive oil to improve pourability (undiluted, it solidifies at room temperature). I add it to insect-repellent spray and solid formulations, as it creates an amazingly effective "bug-blocking aura" around your being — blocking all things that bite from invading your space. I also add the oil to household insecticidal sprays. I use the dried, crushed leaves and powder in bug-repellent sachets and flea- and tick-repellent powder formulations for pets.

PARTS USED: Oil, leaves

ORANGE, SWEET (*Citrus sinensis*)

Sweet orange essential oil and peel have similar insecticidal properties as lemon essential oil and peel.

PARTS USED: Peel, essential oil

SUBSTITUTE: Lemon essential oil and peel; grapefruit essential oil and peel

CAUTIONS: Avoid use of the essential oil if pregnant or epileptic. May be photosensitizing and a potential skin irritant.

PATCHOULI (*Pogostemon cablin*)

This bushy, perennial herb, native to tropical Asia, is often recognized by its pungent, heavy, earthy "hippie era" scent that, while appealing to many humans, effectively wards off spiders, moths, and other creepy-crawlers in your home. The dried leaves and essential oil make great additions to herbal insect-repellent sachets. The leaves can be ground and blended with food-grade diatomaceous earth and used to kill fleas and their larvae lurking on your floors, carpeting, and furniture.

PARTS USED: Essential oil, leaves

PENNYROYAL
(*Mentha pulegium* or *Hedeoma pulegioides*)

Pennyroyal, a strongly aromatic relative of peppermint, is an age-old insecticide with toxic pulegone compounds that kill most insects. When combined with other herbs, it works synergistically to make them more effective at killing or repelling bugs. Pennyroyal is extremely effective at repelling mosquitoes, flies, fleas, ticks, moths, mice, rats, and ants. The dried leaves are used in sachet blends, and either the dried or fresh leaves can be used to make infused oils and tinctures. Powdered leaves can be added to food-grade diatomaceous earth and sprinkled on flooring and furniture.

PART USED: Leaves

PEPPERMINT *(Mentha × piperita)*

A pleasingly pungent, familiar herb, with a biting, minty aroma, peppermint leaves effectively deter moths, ants, and other crawling insects (especially when combined with dried tansy, rosemary, patchouli, cedarwood, pennyroyal, and bay leaves). The essential oil is used in insect repellents for people; to inoculate fabric clothes hangers; in pet shampoos and bedding sachets; as well as in housecleaning and indoor pest-repellent formulations.

PARTS USED: Leaves, essential oil

SUBSTITUTE: Spearmint *(Mentha spicata)* essential oil is somewhat milder but is completely safe to use by pregnant or lactating women, unlike peppermint essential oil.

CAUTION: Avoid using the essential oil if pregnant or epileptic.

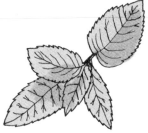

ROSEMARY *(Rosmarinus officinalis)*

A familiar culinary herb with a strong, sharp, camphorous, herbaceous aroma, rosemary contains insect-repellent compounds such as limonene, cineole, and camphor, among others, and effectively repels all manner of insects, especially fleas, ticks, mosquitoes, and flies. The essential oil is derived from the flowering tops and is used in mosquito-repellent formulations; to inoculate fabric clothes hangers; in pet shampoos and on flea collars; and in herbal house-cleaning blends. The dried leaves and essential oil are added to bug-repellent sachets and flea- and tick-repellent powders for flooring, furniture, and pets; also the leaves can be made into a tea and used as a final rinse after shampooing your pet.

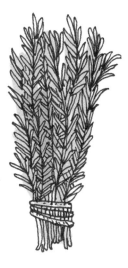

PARTS USED: Leaves, essential oil

SUBSTITUTE: The essential oils of thyme or eucalyptus (species *globulus*, *radiata*, or *smithii*), and leaves of thyme, eucalyptus, basil, or bay may be substituted.

CAUTION: Avoid use of the essential oil if pregnant or epileptic.

SAGE *(Salvia officinalis)*
OR SAGE, SPANISH *(S. lavandulifolia)*

Called *herba sacra* (sacred herb), by the Romans, sage, which is native to the Mediterranean region, is a familiar culinary herb, with a fresh, warm-spicy, herbaceous aroma, often associated with the Thanksgiving holiday. The pale, dusty-green leaves are quite bitter and contain the chemical compounds thujone, camphor, and cineole, making sage quite unappealing to insects of all kinds.

PART USED: Leaves
SUBSTITUTE: Mugwort or wormwood leaves may be substituted for sage leaves.

TANSY (*Tanacetum vulgare*)

A relative of the chrysanthemums and pyrethrums, this pungent, extremely bitter, pretty perennial herb has potent natural insecticidal properties and has been used for centuries to deter bugs. Tansy leaves and flowers contain the chemical constituents thujone, sesquiterpene lactones, pyrethrins, tanacetin, and camphor — all of which are toxic to a wide variety of pests in the home and garden. The leaves and flowers can be utilized in many ways: crushed or ground in bug-repellent sachets or powders; made into a tincture and used as a mosquito-repellent base; or made into a tea and sprayed directly onto areas where bugs are a problem.

PARTS USED: Leaves and flowers
SUBSTITUTE: Feverfew leaves and flowers (*Tanacetum parthenium*)
CAUTION: The fresh plant can irritate skin — so always wear gloves when harvesting.

TEA TREE *(Melaleuca alternifolia)*

Distilled from the leaves and twigs of a small, shrubby tree native to Australia, energetically cooling tea tree essential oil, with its strong, penetrating, medicinal, camphorous odor, and potent anti-inflammatory and antibacterial properties, is an excellent addition to the home medicine cabinet. It is gentle enough to be used "neat" (undiluted) as a spot treatment for hot, itchy insect bites and stings and also has mild-to-moderate bug-repellent properties.

PART USED: Essential oil

THYME *(Thymus vulgaris)*

This familiar culinary herb with a strong, medicinal, slightly sweet, herbaceous aroma, acts as a mild-to-moderately strong repellent against all manner of insects, especially mosquitoes, moths, and fleas. I prefer to use the linalool chemotype of essential oil, derived from the leaves, as it is nontoxic, skin-friendly, gentle, and safe to use on children when properly diluted. Thyme essential oil (either the milder linalool chemotype or hotter thymol chemotype) can also be used in sprays for cleaning counters, bathrooms, and kitchen cabinets. The dried leaves are added to bug-repellent sachets and flea and tick-repellent powders for flooring, furniture, and pets. Additionally, the leaves can be made into a tea and used as a final rinse after shampooing your pet.

PARTS USED: Leaves, essential oil (chemotypes linalool and thymol)
SUBSTITUTE: Fresh lemon thyme herb *(Thymus citriodorus)*, with its potent lemony aroma, can be dried and used in all recipes calling

for regular culinary thyme, as can basil, rosemary, sage, and eucalyptus.

CAUTIONS: Avoid use of the essential oil if pregnant or epileptic. Potential skin irritant.

~~~~~~

VANILLA *(Vanilla planifolia)*

Most people love the intoxicatingly sweet and creamy scent of tropical vanilla beans, which are native to Central America and Mexico. Not everyone knows, however, that vanilla extract (the alcoholic extract of fermented and dried vanilla beans), when combined with other pungent essential oils, works amazingly well at repelling bugs. The principal chemical constituent of vanilla is vanillin aldehyde, which gives it the familiar rich aroma and flavor but also confers mild-to-moderate insect repelling properties.

PART USED: Natural vanilla flavoring (alcohol extract, unsweetened)

~~~~~~

VETIVER *(Vetiveria zizanoides)*

Also known as khus, vetiver is a tall plant, native to India, with grasslike leaves. Vetiver essential oil is derived from the roots, which are strongly scented, reminiscent of an earthy, exotic, smoky blend of sandalwood, violets, grass, and vanilla. Perfumers often use the lingering, heavy aromatic to add a deep note; it also fixes, or stabilizes, the scent. Men tend to find vetiver quite appealing, but moths, silverfish, ants, cockroaches, and many other crawling insects find it quite repulsive.

PART USED: Essential oil

SUBSTITUTE: Dried, chopped vetiver root or root powder, if available, can be added to insect-repellent sachets.

WALNUT, BLACK (*Juglans nigra*)

Intensely bitter and strongly astringent, black walnut hull powder has potent anthelmintic (deworming) and insecticidal properties. It's a good addition to flea- and tick-repellent powder blends for pets, as these pests abhor the flavor and scent of this ingredient.

PART USED: Nut hull powder

WORMWOOD (*Artemisia absinthium*)

Wormwood, a rather pungent, extremely bitter perennial herb with potent insecticidal and vermicidal properties, has been used for centuries, as most household bugs abhor its flavor and fragrance. The leaves contain thujone, absinthol, and camphor, all highly toxic to insect pests in the home and garden. The dried leaves can be used in sachets to repel moths residing in kitchen cabinets, clothes closets, armoires, and drawers, as well as in pet bedding sachets. I use the powdered leaves in flea repellents and insecticidal blends for pets, furniture, and flooring.

PART USED: Leaves
SUBSTITUTE: Mugwort leaves

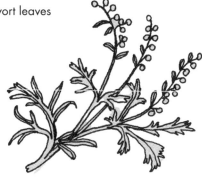

YARROW *(Achillea millefolium)*

This pretty garden herb, with clusters of tiny flowers and small, feathery leaves, is native to Europe and western Asia and naturalized in many regions around the world. Strongly bitter and astringent, with a rather sharp, pungent aroma, yarrow has antiseptic and anti-inflammatory properties, with a cooling energy, and contains insect-repellent chemical compounds such as terpineol, cineole, camphor, and thujone, among others, which bugs hate. I primarily make an herbal tincture from the leaves and flowers, dried or fresh, and use this as a base to which I add essential oils when formulating mosquito-repellent sprays. Additionally, the tincture can be dabbed onto hot, itchy insect bites and stings to quickly cool and calm the irritation. I also add the powdered herb to diatomaceous earth–based flea and tick powders for my cats.

PARTS USED: Leaves and flowers

Make a "Neat" Bug-Repellent Hat

To fend off flying insect attacks during the height of mosquito, blackfly, and deerfly season, many residents of the great state of Maine (where I live) who want to be outdoors — working, hunting, fishing, gardening, camping, hiking, or exercising — will inoculate a hat of any type with a few drops of "neat" or undiluted star anise, citronella, geranium, catnip, rosemary, cedarwood, lemongrass, or eucalyptus essential oil prior to venturing outside. A simple solution, but amazingly effective!

Base Ingredients and Additives

BAKING SODA (SODIUM BICARBONATE)

This white, crystalline, odorless, salty-tasting alkaline powder absorbs moisture and neutralizes odors, making it an excellent addition to herbal insecticide carpet powder blends. Additionally, an application of a baking-soda-and-water paste is an old-fashioned remedy that relieves the pain and itch of most insect bites and bee stings.

BEESWAX

Pure, unrefined, unbleached beeswax is used as a thickener in solid insect-repellent balms and in herbal salves for soothing skin irritated by bites and stings. Beeswax adds a sweet, honey-like aroma and golden color to products. Melted beeswax hardens quickly as it cools. Beeswax is available in several forms: blocks or chunks that can be whacked into smaller pieces; honeycomb sheets that can be broken or cut; or small pellets or pastilles that can be measured and melted with ease. SUBSTITUTE: Refined vegetable emulsifying wax or soybean wax are good vegan options.

BENTONITE CLAY

This naturally occurring volcanic ash, a pale to medium gray powder with a medium-fine texture, is found in the midwestern United States and Canada (the name comes from Benton, Montana). Chock-full of beneficial minerals, including silica, it is used as a base for making herbal flea and tick powders. It interferes with the respiratory systems of these insects and dehydrates their bodies, too.

CAUTION: Though bentonite clay is a nontoxic ingredient, avoid creating a cloud of dust when using it or adding it to a recipe, as it can be slightly irritating to the mucous membranes and respiratory tract.

BORAX (SODIUM BORATE)

Common borax can be found in the laundry aisle of your grocery store — look for 20 Mule Team Borax. It is a white, crystalline mineral, large quantities of which are mined in southern California. Borax has diverse household uses, including as a water softener; cleaning aid; emulsifier; natural preservative and buffering agent in homemade cosmetics; deodorizer; and mold inhibitor. It is frequently used as a natural household insecticide, acting as both a stomach poison to which insects don't become immune and as a desiccant that destroys the waxy coating that protects insects from water loss and subsequent dehydration.

After coming into contact with borax, insects clean themselves, thereby ingesting the powder, leading to death within a few days (or less); that is, if they haven't already succumbed to death by dehydration. It may sound gruesome, but borax is one of the least toxic, most effective, and longest-lasting substances for ridding your home of nearly all creepy-crawly bugs, especially bad infestations of fleas, ants, and cockroaches. To ensure maximum effectiveness, sprinkle it evenly and uniformly all over the surfaces you are treating, or insects will simply gather on untreated areas. Spreading it directly on the insects or placing borax unavoidably in their path is a surefire way to control traffic and potential infestations. For a container, I recycle a large plastic spice jar or poke holes in the metal top of a widemouthed canning jar using a hammer and fat nail. Cleanup is easy — after 24 hours or so, simply vacuum all treated areas thoroughly.

SUBSTITUTE: Food-grade diatomaceous earth (see next page)

CAUTIONS: Borax is toxic if ingested, so store it and products made with it away from children and pets (including birds). Keep children and pets out of rooms being treated with borax until all surfaces are vacuumed. Borax can be highly irritating to the mucous membranes and respiratory tract, so avoid breathing it in. Hold the container close to the treatment surface and sprinkle gently so as not to create dust. A mask and goggles may be worn as a precaution.

CASTILE SOAP, LIQUID

This gentle, olive oil– or hemp oil–based soap is used as a base for herbal dog and cat shampoos — the peppermint and eucalyptus scents work best. (Cats — if you can actually get them to cooperate in a tub of water — prefer milder aromas such as lavender, almond, or unscented baby soap.) Also, liquid castile soap acts as an emulsifier in some of my alcohol- and water-based and witch hazel–based spray repellent formulations, as it helps the essential oils remain in suspension.

COCONUT OIL *(Cocos nucifera)*

Derived from the fruit of the coconut palm, this highly emollient and penetrable, medium-textured, gentle base or carrier oil works well in oil-based formulations that are designed to be rubbed into the skin. Keep in mind that coconut oil is solid at temperatures below 76°F (25°C) and may need to be gently melted before mixing it with other ingredients. Coconut oil is very shelf stable; it requires no refrigeration and will easily last for 2 years if stored in a cool, dark cabinet.

SUBSTITUTE: I use only organic, extra-virgin, unrefined coconut oil because I love the sweet, tropical scent and skin-conditioning properties. You can use refined coconut oil or fractionated coconut oil, but both are devoid of fragrance, flavor, and the raw healing elements contained within the real deal.

FOOD-GRADE DIATOMACEOUS EARTH

Diatomaceous earth (DE) is not actually earth or dirt at all, but fossilized diatom shells ground into powder. Diatoms, a type of one-celled phytoplankton found in both fresh and salt water, form a glasslike protective exterior made from silica. When they die, they sink, resulting in large mineral deposits, often hundreds of feet thick, which are found in abundance worldwide, and harvested as "fossil flour."

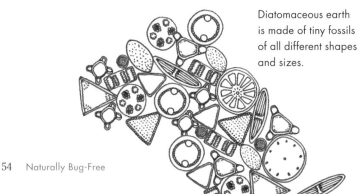

Diatomaceous earth is made of tiny fossils of all different shapes and sizes.

Silica kills mechanically, so insects cannot become immune to its action. It works as a powerful desiccant, leading to dehydration, usually within 24 to 72 hours. Because it is a dust, it also suffocates them. DE is effective against just about any crawling insect, even bedbugs. Many people prefer to use it instead of borax, as it is totally nontoxic to people, pets, and birds. In fact, it acts as a natural and totally safe source of minerals, as well as an effective dewormer, because it does the same thing to internal parasites that it does to external ones.

To ensure maximum effectiveness, sprinkle it evenly on surfaces — and that includes pets — or else the crawling insects will gather on untreated areas. Hold the container a couple of inches above the treatment surface and gently sprinkle the mix to avoid creating a cloud of potentially irritating dust. Dusting directly on the insects or placing DE unavoidably in their path is a surefire way of controlling traffic and potential infestations.

Cleanup is easy — after 24 hours or so, vacuum all treated areas thoroughly, the exception being your pet (though I've known people whose pets enjoyed a good vacuuming, strange as that may sound!). Reapply as often as necessary.

CAUTIONS: Never use "filter-grade" DE, the highly abrasive grade used as a deodorizer and cleaner in aquarium and swimming pool filtering systems. Though derived from the same source as food-grade DE, it is partially dehydrated and chemically treated and extremely irritating to the lungs. For garden, household, and pet use, it must say "food grade" on the label!

GLYCERIN, VEGETABLE

Derived from vegetable fats, this clear, water-soluble, slippery, thickly textured, moisturizing ingredient is added in small amounts to alcohol-based insect repellents in order to moderate the drying effect of the alcohol on the skin.

JOJOBA OIL *(Simmondsia chinensis)*

This light- to medium-textured oil (technically a liquid wax ester) is derived from the seeds of a desert shrub that is cultivated in the southwestern United States, Argentina, and Israel. Chemically similar to human sebum, jojoba oil is a nongreasy, highly penetrable, gentle base or carrier oil I often use in oil-based formulations that are rubbed into the skin. It is preferred by many herbal medicine crafters because it is very shelf-stable; it does not go rancid.

MENTHOL CRYSTALS

Another valuable product of the mint family is menthol crystals, which are derived from the cornmint *(Mentha arvensis)* plant. The slender, quartzlike crystals have an extremely powerful menthol aroma and can be added to sachets to help repel ants, cockroaches, clothing and pantry moths, and other crawling insects, as well as mice. They can also be placed in tiny bags and used in place of toxic, pungent mothballs. Your clothes will smell wonderfully fresh!

CAUTION: Avoid using if pregnant or epileptic. The volatile oils are extremely irritating to the eyes and mucous membranes. Wash hands immediately after working with menthol crystals.

SHEA BUTTER

(*Vitellaria paradoxa,* formerly *Butyrospermum parkii*)

Pressed from the nuts of the karite tree, unrefined shea butter, creamy to pale gold in color with an often distinctive, light, nutty fragrance, is a soft, solid fat that when added to salve and balm formulations contributes a thick and creamy texture, with emollient, skin-softening properties. It takes much longer to harden than beeswax, so keep that in mind when using it as the primary thickening agent. Your product will need additional time to completely set up — sometimes up to 48 hours, depending on the temperature of the room.

SUBSTITUTE: Refined shea butter works just as well but is odorless and white in color and lacks some of the wonderful nutrient qualities of its unrefined cousin.

SOYBEAN OIL (*Glycine max,* syn. *Soja hispida*)

Derived from soybeans, this is a light- to medium-textured, pale gold base or carrier oil with a velvety texture. It is naturally high in vitamin E and lecithin, nongreasy, and easily absorbed into the skin. It has mild insect-repellent properties and is often used in natural oil-based repellents that get rubbed into the skin.

Use only organic soybean oil, as the nonorganic oil (typically labeled "vegetable oil" in the grocery store) is refined at high temperatures and chock-full of chemical residue; also, it is more than likely derived from genetically modified soybeans, and you probably don't want that on your skin. Organic soybean oil has a shelf life of approximately one year if stored in a dark, cool cabinet, but I keep mine in the refrigerator, like most of my edible oils.

SUBSTITUTE: Sunflower seed, jojoba, almond, grapeseed, or apricot kernel oil can be used as substitutes, but they don't deliver the same velvety texture to formulations, nor do they contain the mild insect-repelling properties.

VODKA (ETHYL ALCOHOL)

Typically derived from the fermentation of grain or potatoes, this fragrance-free, clear, antiseptic, alcoholic product is used as an extractive solvent or menstruum when making herbal, alcohol-based tinctures that are used as a spray base for insect repellents for people and insecticides for home use. I also use plain vodka blended with purified water and essential oils for the same purposes. When formulations are applied to the skin, the alcohol evaporates quickly, leaving behind the herb's bug-repelling properties. Always purchase 80- or 100-proof, unsweetened, unflavored vodka; an inexpensive variety is fine.

CAUTION: Avoid applying to dry, irritated, sensitive, burned, or abraded skin, except as indicated by the recipe to treat insect stings and bites in order to prevent future infection.

WITCH HAZEL *(Hamamelis virginiana)*

A small, deciduous tree with petite, bright yellow, stringy flowers, native to the damp woodlands of eastern North America and Nova Scotia, witch hazel has a rather cooling energy with anti-inflammatory, antibacterial, and astringent properties. It contains the chemical compounds eugenol and carvacrol, plus tannins, all of which insects find distasteful. I sometimes use it as the liquid base to which I add essential oils when making insect-repellent sprays. Applied directly to skin, it effectively cools and calms insect bites and stings and helps prevent infection.

PART USED: Commercially prepared liquid

SUBSTITUTE: Tincture of yarrow diluted 50 percent with purified water

CAUTION: Avoid applying to dry, irritated, sensitive, burned, or abraded skin, except as indicated by the recipe to treat insect stings and bites, and to prevent future infection.

Garden-Fresh Insect Repellent

The fresh leaves of catnip, rosemary, thyme (and lemon thyme), eucalyptus, pennyroyal, peppermint, wormwood, mugwort, basil, yarrow (flowers and leaves), and lavender (buds and leaves) can be rubbed directly onto your skin to provide a temporary, light-to-moderately effective, insect-repelling aura. (Dogs and cats can benefit from a rubdown as well.) 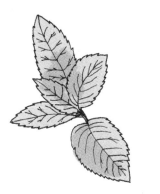 **Note:** If your skin becomes red or itches after applying fresh herbs in this manner, wash immediately with warm, soapy water to remove the plant's oils.

Chapter 3

MIXING IT UP:
ESSENTIAL
EQUIPMENT

A Few Tools of the Trade

Anything you need should be readily available at your local home goods, department, kitchenware, or hardware store or from online purveyors of related kitchen equipment. Here's a list of the basics.

BLENDER, COFFEE GRINDER, OR FOOD PROCESSOR. I primarily use a blender to pulverize dried herb matter such as flowers, buds, and leaves to near powder consistency, though it's not suitable for really tough herbs such as dried roots, bark, or twigs. A food processor also works well, as does a coffee grinder, though the coffee grinder will grind only small amounts.

BOWLS. You'll need a variety of sizes in glass, enamel, plastic, stainless steel, or ceramic. Copper or aluminum can react adversely with some of the chemical compounds in the herbs and essential oils.

Keep It Clean

"Cleanliness is next to godliness," as the saying goes, and whether you're preparing dinner for eight or crafting natural products for personal, pet, or home use, the same sanitary precautions apply. I'm a stickler about proper sanitation. Prior to use, every implement, piece of equipment, or storage container should be run through the dishwasher or washed in very hot soapy water and allowed to air-dry, upside down, on a rack. You don't want to introduce bacteria into your newly made herbal products by using dirty tools or storage containers! Thoroughly clean and dry all your utensils after using them, as well.

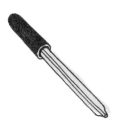

DROPPER (GLASS). Sometimes called an eyedropper, these are used for measuring essential oils by the drop. Glass is preferable to plastic because it doesn't retain scent or color from the oils, and some essential oils, especially citrus oils, will rapidly degrade plastic and rubber. After each use, rinse the dropper with hot water, then pour isopropyl rubbing alcohol or 95 percent ethyl alcohol (inexpensive 80-proof vodka works great) through it to sterilize it.

Most essential oils come in small, 10-milliliter or 15-milliliter bottles, with "drop-by-drop" reducers for easy application, eliminating the need for a dropper, but larger bottles are often sealed with a simple screw top.

FUNNEL. A small one made of plastic or stainless steel makes it easier to pour liquids into narrow-necked storage bottles.

MEASURING CUPS AND SPOONS. Glass, plastic, or stainless-steel cups and spoons used for baking are fine.

POTS/PANS. For making balms and infused oils, I use several sizes, from 2 cups to 2 quarts, made of enamel, glass, or stainless steel. Don't use aluminum or copper, which can react with the chemical compounds in the herbs.

SPATULAS. Collect a variety of sizes for scooping out balms, salves, shea butter, and wet clay from any type of container. Short, narrow spatulas are useful for filling small jars with thickened salves and balms or for transferring products from one container to another.

SPOONS AND STIRRING UTENSILS. One small and one medium wooden spoon are indispensable. A stainless steel iced-tea spoon works well for blending liquids in tiny pans or if you don't have a short, narrow wooden spoon handy. Wooden chopsticks, ½-inch-diameter dowels, and the handles of wooden spoons are useful for poking into tall containers, as well as for dredging sludgy oil- or alcohol-sodden herbs from the bottom of saucepans or canning jars. A basic, medium-size whisk of any material works well for blending batches of powders containing powdered ingredients and essential oils.

STRAINERS. Bamboo, wire, or fabric mesh — use them to strain herbs from liquids when making teas, infused oils, and tinctures (alcohol extracts) or to support finer filters when straining smaller particles.

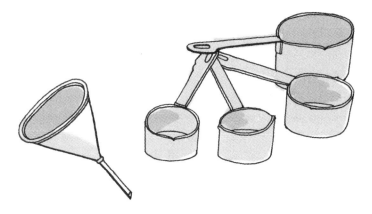

Storage Containers

I like containers that are aesthetically pleasing, but it's more important to select ones that are appropriate for the product, such as a shaker container for flea or carpet powders, a spritzer bottle for sprays, and muslin bags or large custom-brew tea bags for potpourri blends used to deter moths and other insects.

Many retailers carry suitable containers. Check with arts and crafts suppliers, hardware stores, home goods (kitchen, bed, and bath) stores, herb shops, larger health food stores, and grocers that cater to healthy lifestyles. If you can't find what you want locally, search the Internet. As always, buying in bulk saves money. Sharing the container order with a friend or two saves money as well. I generally purchase containers by the dozen from mail-order bottle companies and a few of my favorite large, mail-order herb shops (Resources, page 170).

Label, Label, Label!

Always label your creations with the list of ingredients and the date it was made and the words "For External Use Only." Any type of label is fine, but because they may get wet and dirty, protect them with clear shipping tape or laminating sheets. I like to give my formulas catchy customized names, such as "Bandit's Bug Bomb Powder" and "Lilly's No-Fleas-on-Me Spray" — these were specially made for my two cats.

BOTTLES. Glass or plastic versions in sizes from 2 to 16 ounces are great for storing and applying liquids. Dark glass — amber or cobalt blue are the most readily available — helps preserve the volatile properties of herbs and oils against the damaging effect of bright light.

CANNING JARS. These clear glass jars come in a variety of sizes and are suitable for storing extracts, infused oils, and tinctures, as well as powdered clay, borax, diatomaceous earth, dried herbs, and large batches of finished formulations.

CREAM JARS. Perfect for storing thick insect-repellent balms, these are available in clear or opaque plastic, or clear, amber, or cobalt blue glass. They come in sizes from ¼ ounce to 8 ounces. You can recycle small condiment jars or baby food jars (washed and sterilized with labels removed), but make sure the lids fit snugly. Store clear jars away from light.

MUSLIN BAGS. Available in a variety of sizes, these are useful for making sachets.

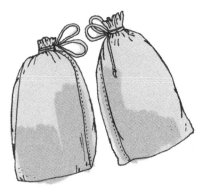

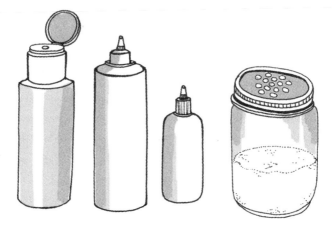

SHAKER CONTAINERS. Large plastic culinary herb containers, the kind with an inner lid full of holes, are perfect for dispensing herbal powders. Glass containers are harder to find, but nice to have. Classic cardboard cylinder shakers are usually sold through herbal mail-order suppliers. Or turn a widemouthed canning jar into a shaker container by poking holes in the metal top.

SPRITZER BOTTLES. These are must-have packaging for any recipe that requires a spray application. Spritzer bottles made of glass or plastic are available in 1-, 2-, 4-, and 8-ounce sizes; 16-ounce bottles are generally made of plastic. Plastic hairspray and hair gel bottles can be recycled for this purpose, if you wish, but must be thoroughly washed out.

SQUEEZE BOTTLES. These plastic bottles, the kind used for personal care products or condiments, are great storage containers for pet shampoos, and alcohol- or oil-based insect repellents.

TEA BAGS (SEAL-AND-BREW, LARGE). These 4-inch by 5-inch, natural-fiber bags are traditionally used for brewing loose-leaf tea, but crafters often use them as herbal sachet pouches instead of the drawstring muslin bags. You simply stuff the tea bag with your herbal bug-repelling blend and press an iron along the open end to seal.

TINS. In sizes of ¼-ounce and up, they're perfect for storing dried herbs, large batches of flea and tick powder and herbal sachet blends, and dry ingredients such as bentonite clay and food-grade diatomaceous earth. Tiny tins make good containers for solid repellent balms.

ZIPLOCK FREEZER BAGS. Herbs are best stored in tightly sealed jars or tins, but ziplock freezer bags are a reasonable and inexpensive alternative, and they're fine for borax, baking soda, clay, diatomaceous earth, and other dry ingredients. If you do use them to store herbs, keep them in a very dry, cool, dark place and use the herbs within a year. **Note:** The slide-lock freezer bags are not airtight; use the double-zipper style instead.

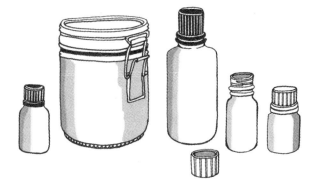

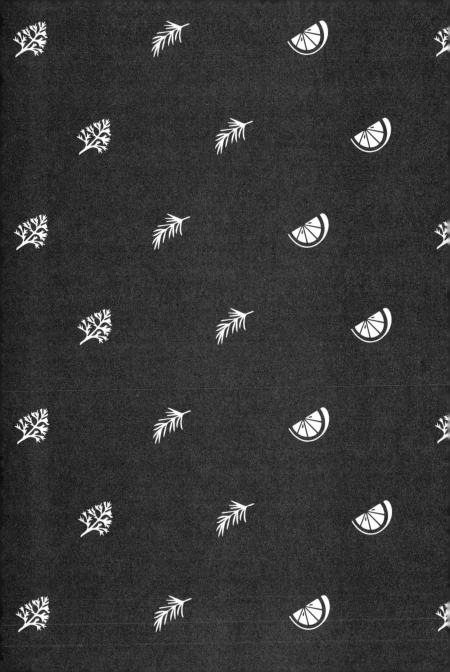

Recipes

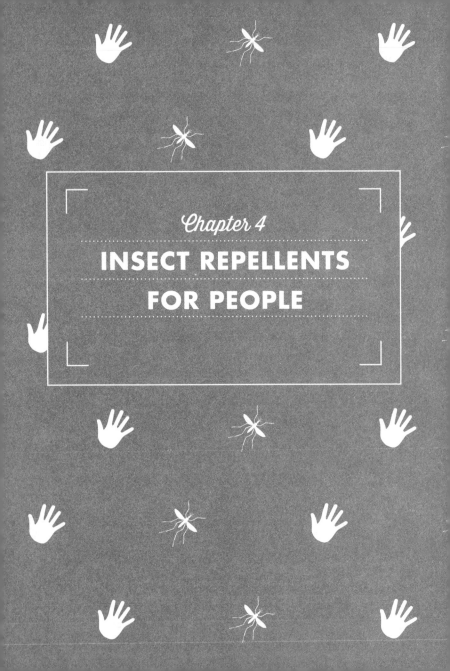

Chapter 4
INSECT REPELLENTS
FOR PEOPLE

The amount of annoyance, discomfort, and disease inflicted by some of the smallest creatures on the planet is astounding — and on a personal scale, often maddening. Instead of reaching for smelly, chemical-based sprays or lotions to fend off pests, keep them at bay with natural, nontoxic products that smell pleasant. These formulations contain strongly aromatic herbs that have been used historically to effectively repel insects. They're totally safe applied to skin or clothing when used as directed, but everyone's body chemistry is unique, so if the first one you make doesn't work as well as you'd like, try another recipe.

Commonsense Safety

- Keep all homemade insect repellent products out of reach of children and pets.

- Use only as directed.

- Don't spray or rub any product directly into your eyes, nose, or mouth or take internally.

- If skin irritation occurs, wash with soap and water, then apply plain cooking oil, calendula or comfrey salve, or zinc-based diaper rash ointment. If irritation persists, seek medical help.

Liquid and Spray Formulations

MOSQUITO FORMULA #1

Oil-based: This formulation can safely be used by pregnant and lactating women, children three years of age and older, and individuals with super-sensitive skin. Its delicate floral-green fragrance appeals to everyone except bugs. This version uses oil as the base ingredient, which leaves skin feeling velvety soft and nongreasy. I like organic soybean oil for its natural bug-repellent properties, but you can substitute any lightweight base oil. For a lighter formulation, choose Formula #2.

Caution: Use one of the two species of eucalyptus essential oils specified. Do not use other species of eucalyptus.

....

16 drops each of the following essential oils: lavender, geranium, eucalyptus (species *radiata* or *smithii*)

½ cup organic soybean base oil
4-ounce spritzer, pump, or squeeze bottle

....

1. Add the lavender, geranium, and eucalyptus essential oils to the storage bottle, then add the soybean oil. Screw the top on the bottle and shake vigorously to blend. Allow the spray to synergize for 1 hour.

2. Store at room temperature, away from heat and light; use within 1 year.

Application: Shake well before using. Put a bit of this formula on your palms, then massage it onto areas that need protection. If your skin feels greasy after application, you've used too much. Reapply as needed.

MOSQUITO FORMULA #2

Alcohol-and-water-based: This is the same basic formulation as #1, but uses water and alcohol as a base for a lighter-textured product, which some people prefer, especially in hot, humid climates.

Caution: To ensure gentleness and safety, you must use one of the two species of eucalyptus essential oils specified. Do not use other species of eucalyptus.

....

16 drops each of the following essential oils: lavender, geranium, eucalyptus (species *radiata* or *smithii*)

½ teaspoon liquid castile soap, peppermint or eucalyptus scented

½ teaspoon vegetable glycerin
¼ cup purified water
¼ cup unflavored vodka
4-ounce spritzer bottle

....

1. Add the lavender, geranium, and eucalyptus essential oils directly to the storage bottle, then add the liquid soap, glycerin, water, and vodka. Screw the top on the bottle and shake vigorously to blend. Allow the solution to synergize for 1 hour.

2. Store at room temperature, away from heat and light; use within 1 year.

Application: Shake well before using. Spray liberally onto skin as needed — you may need to reapply it every 20 to 30 minutes. May be sprayed on clothing.

DON'T BE A MOSQUITO MAGNET

3 Ways to Guarantee Fewer Bites

Why do some people seem to attract clouds of bloodthirsty mosquitoes while others can sit around on the back deck all evening with nary a bite? These lucky people apparently don't have the right combination of visual and aromatic "bait." Mosquitoes use their senses to choose tasty targets, so here are some suggestions to make yourself less appetizing.

Keep Clean

The stronger you smell, the easier it is for a hungry mosquito to find you, so shower often and try to stay cool and dry. Ever wonder why mosquitoes seem to target your ankles? They're attracted to the aroma of stinky feet, so change your socks daily. Mosquitoes are also attracted to movement. If you're running around, they'll deem you worthy of an investigation even if they can't smell you yet.

Check your breath, too. Mosquitoes detect the carbon dioxide we exhale and they are drawn to ethanol fumes, so having a couple of drinks at the neighborhood barbecue might lure them to you. Using peppermint mouthwash or essential oil drops to freshen your breath might steer them away.

Stay Neutral

Biting insects seem to be attracted to the same scents that we like, so avoid fragranced personal care products such as soaps, shaving cream, deodorant, hair products, and even laundry detergent. Choose unscented versions and skip the perfume or aftershave if you're planning to be outside during bug season.

Lactic acid is a big draw for mosquitoes, so consider cutting down on yogurt, milk, and cheese. Your body naturally produces lactic acid, but when you eat dairy products, you excrete more of it, making you more desirable. Avoiding skincare products with alpha hydroxy acids might help as well, as many of them contain lactic acid, which is touted to improve the texture and tone of your skin.

Dress for the Occasion

Mosquitoes respond most to dark colors, especially blue and brown, so wear light-colored clothing with loose, long sleeves. Linen provides protection against munching marauders while allowing you to maintain a stylishly cool demeanor.

CHILD'S PLAY SPRAY

Young children are not little adults — they cannot tolerate the concentration of essential oils in strong formulations. This spray is designed for children one year of age and older. It has a pleasing aroma that's wonderfully effective at keeping mildly to moderately hungry biting bugs at bay. When bugs are voracious, clothe children appropriately and inoculate their clothes with a few spritzes. Never "drown" their bare skin in bug spray, even an all-natural one, in an attempt to keep bugs away.

Cautions: To ensure gentleness and safety, you must use one of the two species of eucalyptus essential oils specified as well as the linalool chemotype of thyme. Other varieties of eucalyptus or thyme may irritate the skin.

....

3 drops each of the following essential oils: eucalyptus (species *radiata* or *smithii*), cedarwood, rosemary, lemongrass, thyme (chemotype linalool)

½ **teaspoon** neem base oil

½ **teaspoon** liquid castile soap, peppermint or eucalyptus scented

½ **teaspoon** vegetable glycerin

½ **cup** unflavored vodka

½ **cup** purified water

8-ounce spritzer bottle

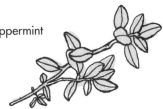

....

1. Add the eucalyptus, cedarwood, rosemary, lemongrass, and thyme essential oils directly to the storage bottle, then add the neem oil, liquid soap, glycerin, vodka, and water. Screw the top on the bottle and shake vigorously to blend. Allow the spray to synergize for 1 hour.

2. Store at room temperature, away from heat and light; use within 1 year.

Application: Shake well immediately before use. Spray lightly onto skin as needed — you may need to reapply it every 20 to 30 minutes. May be sprayed on clothing but might stain light-colored fabrics.

BUG BOGGLE FORMULA #1

Oil-based: I've had this formulation in my herbal remedy recipe box for years. It works wonderfully well with my personal chemistry, and the aroma is quite pleasing, but the bugs apparently don't like it! This version uses oil as the base ingredient, which leaves the skin feeling velvety soft and nongreasy, but if you'd rather use a lighter formulation, make Formula #2, which uses alcohol and water as the base ingredients.

Note: Soybean oil is used as a base for its natural bug-repellent properties, but you can substitute your favorite lightweight, organic base oil such as jojoba, sunflower, grapeseed, or almond.

. . . .

15 drops geranium essential oil
8 drops cedarwood essential oil
8 drops catnip essential oil
6 drops eucalyptus essential oil
6 drops rosemary essential oil

5 drops peppermint essential oil
½ cup organic soybean base oil
4-ounce spritzer, pump, or
    squeeze bottle

. . . .

1. Add the geranium, cedarwood, catnip, eucalyptus, rosemary, and peppermint essential oils directly to the storage bottle, then add the soybean oil. Screw the top on the bottle and shake vigorously to blend. Allow the spray to synergize for 1 hour.

2. Store at room temperature, away from heat and light; use within 1 year.

Application: Shake the bottle prior to each use. I like to put a bit of this formula onto my palms, then massage the oil into areas that need bug protection. It is designed to penetrate quickly. If your skin feels greasy after application, you've used too much. Reapply as needed.

BUG BOGGLE FORMULA #2

Alcohol-and-water-based: This is the same basic formulation as above, but instead of using oil as the base or carrier ingredient, I use a blend of alcohol and water. This combination of ingredients results in a lighter-textured product, which some people prefer, especially in hot, humid climates.

....

15 drops geranium essential oil
8 drops cedarwood essential oil
8 drops catnip essential oil
6 drops eucalyptus essential oil
6 drops rosemary essential oil
5 drops peppermint essential oil

½ **teaspoon** liquid castile soap, peppermint or eucalyptus scented
½ **teaspoon** vegetable glycerin
¼ **cup** purified water
¼ **cup** unflavored vodka
4-ounce spritzer bottle

....

1. Add the geranium, cedarwood, catnip, eucalyptus, rosemary, and peppermint essential oils directly to the storage bottle, then add the liquid soap, glycerin, water, and vodka. Screw the top on the bottle and shake vigorously to blend. Allow the solution to synergize for 1 hour.
2. Store at room temperature, away from heat and light; use within 1 year.

Application: Shake well immediately before use. Spray liberally onto skin as needed — you may need to reapply it every 20 to 30 minutes. May be sprayed on clothing.

LAVENDER LOVER'S INSECT ARMOR

The essential oils in this recipe are exactly the same as those in Essential Tick-Repellent Clothing Drops (page 98), but for this formula, I've diluted them with witch hazel to form a tough-on-bugs, gentle-on-skin, cooling spray with a fragrance that will appeal to lavender lovers everywhere.

. . . .

4 drops each of the following essential oils: catnip, geranium, and peppermint
1¼ teaspoons lavender essential oil (approximately 125 drops)
½ teaspoon liquid castile soap, peppermint or eucalyptus scented
½ teaspoon vegetable glycerin
1 cup witch hazel
8-ounce spritzer bottle

. . . .

1. Add the catnip, geranium, peppermint, and lavender essential oils directly to the storage bottle, then add the liquid soap, glycerin, and witch hazel. Screw the top on the bottle and shake vigorously to blend. Allow the spray to synergize for 1 hour.
2. Store at room temperature, away from heat and light; use within 1 year.

Application: Shake the bottle prior to each use. Apply liberally to skin as needed — you may need to reapply it every 20 to 30 minutes. May be sprayed on clothing.

ROSEMARY & LEMONGRASS INSECT-REPELLENT SPRITZER

This aromatically refreshing blend of two of nature's most potent insect-repelling essential oils will appeal to your sense of smell, but bugs will find you rather offensive.

....

40 drops rosemary essential oil
20 drops lemongrass essential oil
½ teaspoon vegetable glycerin
1 cup witch hazel
8-ounce spritzer bottle

....

1. Add the rosemary and lemongrass essential oils directly to the bottle, then add the glycerin and witch hazel. Screw the top on the bottle and shake vigorously to blend. Allow the spritzer to synergize for 1 hour.
2. Store at room temperature, away from heat and light; use within 1 year.

Application: Shake the bottle prior to each use. Apply liberally to skin as needed — you may need to reapply it every 20 to 30 minutes. May be sprayed on clothing.

LEMON, CEDAR & THYME SPRAY

Oh my, does this repellent smell fabulous — light woodsy-green with the zing of lemon. Even better, this formula is a terrific odor-busting underarm and foot deodorant, as well as a gentle yet powerful home insecticide spray! How's that for a multiuse product?

....

40 drops cedarwood essential oil
20 drops thyme (chemotype linalool) essential oil
15 drops lemon essential oil
½ **teaspoon** vegetable glycerin
1 cup unflavored vodka
Rind of 1 lemon, cut into long, thin strips
8-ounce spritzer bottle

....

1. Add the cedarwood, thyme, and lemon essential oils directly to the bottle, then add the glycerin, vodka, and lemon rind. Screw the top on the bottle and shake vigorously to blend. Allow the spray to synergize for 1 hour. You may leave the rind in the bottle for up to 1 month, then remove.
2. Store at room temperature, away from heat and light; use within 1 year.

Application: Shake the bottle prior to each use. Apply liberally to skin as needed — you may need to reapply every 20 to 30 minutes. May be sprayed on clothing.

LEMONY EUCALYPTUS-GERANIUM TICK-REPELLENT SPRAY

When these four essential oils — lemon eucalyptus, geranium, lemongrass, and citronella — are combined, the result is a potent, safe, and pleasingly aromatic tick repellent that works wonderfully well at fending off flying insects, too.

Note: You can substitute *Eucalyptus globulus* essential oil, if *E. citriodora* is unavailable. The formula will still be effective, but the lemon aroma will be lighter.

....

20 drops geranium essential oil

14 drops lemon eucalyptus essential oil

7 drops lemongrass essential oil

7 drops citronella essential oil

½ **teaspoon** liquid castile soap, peppermint or eucalyptus scented

½ **teaspoon** vegetable glycerin

¼ **cup** purified water

¼ **cup** unflavored vodka

4-ounce spritzer bottle

....

1. Add the geranium, lemon eucalyptus, lemongrass, and citronella essential oils directly to the storage bottle, then add the liquid soap, glycerin, water, and vodka. Screw the top on the bottle and shake vigorously to blend. Allow the spray to synergize for 1 hour.

2. Store at room temperature, away from heat and light; use within 1 year.

Application: Shake well immediately before use. Spray liberally onto skin as needed — you may need to reapply every 20 to 30 minutes. May stain light-colored fabrics.

LEMONY BUGS-AWAY SPRAY

This light-textured, rather mild repellent leaves your skin feeling fresh and clean and scented with a lingering, lemony aroma generally enjoyed by all. Originally published in my best-selling book, *Organic Body Care Recipes*, this recipe has always been quite popular with readers who like a light, lemon-scented spray, so I thought I'd share it here.

....

2 cups witch hazel
1 teaspoon vegetable glycerin
20 drops citronella essential oil

20 drops lemongrass essential oil
16-ounce spritzer bottle or several
  smaller bottles

....

1. Combine the witch hazel, glycerin, citronella essential oil, and lemongrass essential oil in a 16-ounce bottle. Shake vigorously to blend. Allow the solution to synergize for 1 hour. Decant into several smaller spritzer bottles if desired.
2. Store at room temperature, away from heat and light; use within 1 year.

Application: Shake the bottle prior to each use. Apply liberally to skin as needed — you may need to reapply every 20 minutes. May stain light-colored fabrics.

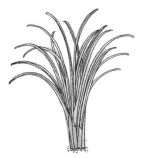

BYE, BYE, BUZZY SPRAY

If you love the uplifting, stimulating scents of rosemary, lemon, and peppermint, then you'll adore this mentally energizing formula that happens to repel annoying bugs. It doubles as a wonderfully effective, antiseptic kitchen and bathroom cleaner, leaving a lingering fragrance that will help deter all manner of pesky insects, especially in dark cabinets where they like to reside.

....

40 drops rosemary essential oil
30 drops lemon essential oil
10 drops peppermint essential oil
½ teaspoon vegetable glycerin

½ teaspoon liquid castile soap, peppermint or eucalyptus scented
1 cup witch hazel
8-ounce spritzer bottle

....

1. Add the rosemary, lemon, and peppermint essential oils directly to the bottle, then add the glycerin, liquid soap, and witch hazel. Screw the top on the bottle and shake vigorously to blend. Allow the spray to synergize for 1 hour.
2. Store at room temperature, away from heat and light; use within 1 year.

Application: Shake the bottle prior to each use. Apply liberally to skin as needed — you may need to reapply every 20 to 30 minutes. May be sprayed on clothing.

OUTDOOR REPELLENT SMUDGE

Powdered mugwort is the main ingredient used in the man-ufacturing of moxa sticks, the long, slender, cigar-size sticks that are used in the traditional Chinese medicine therapy called moxibustion. I purchase these in bulk from Chinese herbal supply houses and burn them as insect-repellent incense sticks when enjoying a warm evening out on my back deck or while camping. They work like a charm and seem-ingly burn forever!

You can make your own herbal smudge based on dried mugwort, which has an easily ignited, cottony consistency. Combine it in a one-to-one ratio with another dried herb such as rosemary, culinary or white sage, lavender buds, or cedar leaves (1½ teaspoons of mugwort for each 1½ teaspoons of the other herb). Burn a tablespoon of the mixture at a time over a piece of incense charcoal in a seashell or other shal-low, suitable container. The fragrant smoke effectively repels mosquitoes, gnats, no-see-ums, biting flies, and bees from your immediate outdoor surroundings. For maximum bug-repellent power, place several smudge bowls around your dining area. Interesting to note, the smoke from any of these herbs, alone or in combination, was (and still is) traditionally used to purify the physical and spiritual environment.

SUMMER THYME REPELLENT #1

Oil-based: A winning combination of some of nature's most powerful insect-repelling herbs, this is one of my stronger formulations. Give it a try if other herbal blends haven't worked for you. Its rather pungent fragrance creates an amazingly effective aura that masks your personal scent. Bugs will find you most unappealing and seek tastier flesh. This version uses oil as the base ingredient, which leaves the skin feeling velvety soft, but if you'd rather a lighter product, make Repellent #2, which uses alcohol and water as the base ingredients.

Note: Soybean oil is used as a base for its natural bug-repellent properties, but you can substitute your favorite organic base oil such as jojoba, sunflower, grapeseed, or almond.

....

10 drops lemongrass essential oil
6 drops thyme (chemotype linalool) essential oil
6 drops rosemary essential oil
4 drops catnip essential oil

½ teaspoon neem base oil
½ cup organic soybean base oil
4-ounce spritzer, pump, or squeeze bottle

....

1. Add the lemongrass, thyme, rosemary, and catnip essential oils directly to the bottle, then add the neem and soybean oils. Screw the top on the bottle and shake vigorously to blend. Allow the oil to synergize for 1 hour.
2. Store at room temperature, away from heat and light; use within 1 year.

Application: Shake well before using. Put a bit of oil onto your palms, then massage into areas that need bug protection. If your skin feels greasy after application, you've used too much. Reapply as needed.

SUMMER THYME REPELLENT #2

Alcohol-and-water-based: This is the same basic formulation as #1, but made with a blend of alcohol and water instead of oil as the carrier. This results in a lighter-textured product, which some people prefer, especially in hot, humid climates.

....

10 drops lemongrass essential oil
6 drops thyme (chemotype linalool) essential oil
6 drops rosemary essential oil
4 drops catnip essential oil
½ teaspoon neem base oil

½ teaspoon liquid castile soap, peppermint or eucalyptus scented
½ teaspoon vegetable glycerin
¼ cup purified water
¼ cup unflavored vodka
4-ounce spritzer bottle

....

1. Add the lemongrass, thyme, rosemary, and catnip essential oils directly to the bottle. Next, add the neem oil, liquid soap, glycerin, water, and vodka. Screw the top on the bottle and shake vigorously to blend. Allow the spray to synergize for 1 hour.
2. Store at room temperature, away from heat and light; use within 1 year.

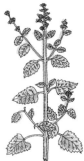

Application: Shake well before using. Spray liberally onto skin as needed — approximately every 20 to 40 minutes. May stain light-colored fabrics.

SWAT-NO-MORE!

Enjoy the outdoors without having to shoo away and slap at all those annoying flying insects, not to mention the itching and scratching that follow. This simple, skin-friendly repellent spray with a light, nutty-green scent works wonders. Kids and teens love it!

. . . .

20 drops eucalyptus essential oil (species *globulus, radiata*, or *smithii*)

15 drops geranium essential oil

15 drops rosemary essential oil

10 drops lavender essential oil

6 drops peppermint essential oil

4 drops catnip essential oil

½ **teaspoon** neem base oil

½ **teaspoon** liquid castile soap, peppermint or eucalyptus scented

½ **teaspoon** vegetable glycerin

1 cup witch hazel

8-ounce spritzer bottle

. . . .

1. Add the eucalyptus, geranium, rosemary, lavender, peppermint, and catnip essential oils directly to the bottle, then add the neem oil, liquid soap, glycerin, and witch hazel. Screw the top on the bottle and shake vigorously to blend. Allow the spray to synergize for 1 hour.

2. Store at room temperature, away from heat and light; use within 1 year.

Application: Shake the bottle prior to each use. Apply liberally to skin as needed — approximately every 30 minutes. May stain light-colored fabrics.

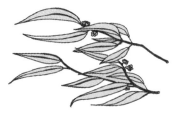

VANILLA–STAR ANISE SPICE SPRAY

This insect repellent has an unexpected warm, spicy sweet vanilla-licorice-lemon scent — almost like spiced candy! It's favored by kids and adults alike, but not by bugs.

....

20 drops lemongrass essential oil
14 drops star anise essential oil
2 drops clove essential oil
2 drops cinnamon bark essential oil
½ teaspoon vegetable glycerin

1 tablespoon natural vanilla extract (alcohol based, unsweetened)
3 tablespoons unflavored vodka
¼ cup purified water
4-ounce spritzer bottle

....

1. Add the lemongrass, star anise, clove, and cinnamon bark essential oils directly to the bottle, then add the glycerin, vanilla extract, vodka, and water. Screw the top on the bottle and shake vigorously to blend. Allow the spray to synergize for 1 hour.

2. Store at room temperature, away from heat and light; use within 1 year.

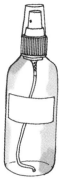

Application: Shake well immediately before use. Spray liberally onto skin as needed — approximately every 20 to 30 minutes. May be sprayed on clothing but might stain light-colored fabrics.

SKEETER SHIELD

Few people realize that mosquitoes rely on sugar as their main source of energy. Both male and female mosquitoes feed primarily on plant nectar, fruit juice, and liquids that ooze from plants, but only female mosquitoes bite, because they need a blood meal to produce eggs. This trio of sensory-stimulating, powerfully aromatic herbs provides a strong shield against determined hordes. The menthol crystals create a wonderful cooling sensation that is rather nice on a hot day!

Caution: Avoid contact with nose, eyes, and mouth. Wash hands with soap and water immediately after handling menthol crystals.

....

30 drops rosemary essential oil   ½ **teaspoon** vegetable glycerin
18 drops catnip essential oil   **1 cup** unflavored vodka
½ **teaspoon** menthol crystals   8-ounce spritzer bottle

....

1. Add the rosemary and catnip essential oils directly to the bottle, then add the menthol crystals, vegetable glycerin, and vodka. Screw the top on the bottle and shake vigorously to blend.

2. Allow the spray to synergize for 1 hour. **Note:** The menthol crystals will take approximately 20 minutes or more to dissolve in the alcohol. The more you shake, the quicker they break down. If they do not break down completely, that's okay; they will still lend their strong, minty essence to the repellent.

3. Store at room temperature, away from heat and light; use within 1 year.

Application: Shake well before using. Spray liberally onto skin as needed — every 20 to 30 minutes. May be sprayed on clothing.

"DAZED & CONFUSED" ESSENTIAL OIL SPRAY

If you're an aromatherapy fan with a large collection of essential oils, then this formula will probably appeal to you. It contains 12 different oils with a broad spectrum of insect-deterring aromas — sharp, green, spicy, earthy, minty, woody, citrusy, grassy, floral, and medicinal. Such a combination is bound to daze and confuse the most determined blood-sucking insect and send it on its dizzy way!

8 drops each:
   lemongrass essential oil
   cedarwood essential oil
   rosemary essential oil
   eucalyptus essential oil

6 drops each:
   geranium essential oil
   lavender essential oil
   catnip essential oil

4 drops each:
   citronella essential oil
   thyme essential oil

2 drops each:
   tea tree essential oil
   clove essential oil
   lemon essential oil

½ **teaspoon** vegetable glycerin

½ **teaspoon** liquid castile soap, peppermint or eucalyptus scented

¼ **cup** purified water

¾ **cup** unflavored vodka

8-ounce spritzer bottle

1. Add all the essential oils directly to the bottle, then add the vegetable glycerin, liquid soap, water, and vodka. Screw the top on the bottle and shake vigorously to blend. Allow the spray to synergize for 1 hour.
2. Store at room temperature, away from heat and light; use within 1 year.

Application: Shake well immediately before use. Spray liberally onto skin as needed — approximately every 20 to 30 minutes. May be sprayed on clothing.

Balms and Oils

FRESH-SCENT BUG BALM #1

Love the fragrance of rosemary, peppermint, and eucalyptus? Then this solid repellent balm is for you. It conditions your skin while making you smell oh-so-fresh. Everyone around you will find your herbal aroma appealing, but the annoying bugs won't. It's convenient to carry and spillproof, too!

4 tablespoons shea butter (refined or unrefined)
12 drops rosemary essential oil
10 drops eucalyptus essential oil
8 drops peppermint essential oil
Small saucepan; stirring utensil; 2-ounce jar or tin

....

1. Warm the shea butter in the saucepan over low heat until just melted. Remove from the heat, and allow to cool for 5 minutes. Add the rosemary, eucalyptus, and peppermint essential oils, and stir a few times. Pour into storage container, cap, and set aside until the balm has thickened.

2. Unlike beeswax, shea butter can take a long time to completely thicken, and this formula may need up to 24 hours, depending on the temperature. When ready, it will be very thick, semi-hard, and white (or creamy yellow if you use unrefined shea butter).

3. Store at room temperature, away from heat and light; use within 1 year.

Application: If wearing long sleeves and long pants, dab a little on any entry point for biting bugs, such as wrists and ankles, as well as on temples, earlobes, nape of neck, and top of head. If wearing shorts and short sleeves, also apply a very light coating to bare arms and legs. Reapply as needed.

FRESH-SCENT BUG BALM #2

This formula keeps skin-loving shea butter as the base, but these bug-deterring essential oils lend a floral-lemony scent. Follow the instructions for Fresh-Scent Bug Balm #1, substituting these essential oils.

....

4 tablespoons shea butter (refined or unrefined)
20 drops lavender essential oil
15 drops lemongrass essential oil
10 drops citronella essential oil

LAVENDER ICE: MENTHOLATED HEALING OIL

This skin-soothing and calming recipe, first published in my book *Hands-On Healing Remedies*, was originally developed to help heal bruised skin, but it also works amazingly well to comfort skin irritated by bug bites and stings, so I've included it here. The combination of anti-inflammatory, antibacterial lavender essential oil and ultracool cornmint-derived menthol crystals quickly soothes and reduces painful swelling, itchiness, and potential infection. This is strong but gentle medicine: your skin will feel quite chilled upon application, which is a good thing!

Caution: This is an aromatherapeutically concentrated formula. Use by the drop only as directed. Avoid contact with the mucous membranes — the nose, eyes, and mouth. Wash hands immediately after handling menthol crystals.

3 tablespoons plus 1 teaspoon organic soybean, jojoba, sunflower, grapeseed, or almond base oil

2 teaspoons menthol crystals

30 drops lavender essential oil

Small saucepan; stirring utensil; 2-ounce dark glass bottle with dropper top or screw cap

1. Combine the oil and menthol crystals in the saucepan over low heat. Gently warm the mixture just until the crystals dissolve. Remove from the heat. Stir a few times to blend the mixture thoroughly. Pour into a storage bottle and add the lavender essential oil. Screw the top on the bottle, then shake vigorously for 2 minutes to blend. Allow the oil to synergize for 1 hour.

2. Store at room temperature, away from heat and light; use within 1 year.

Application: Shake well before using. Gently massage 1 drop into each insect bite. Repeat three or four times per day for 2 days, or until the itching, heat, and swelling subside. Wash your hands after each application, unless treatment is intended for your fingers or hands, in which case I recommend wearing cotton gloves while the oil soaks in so that you don't unintentionally rub your eyes or nose with the formula.

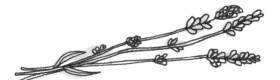

How Often to Apply Natural Repellents

Everyone's experience with the effectiveness of these formulations will vary. My observation has been that natural repellents may need to be reapplied as often as every 20 to 30 minutes, but that depends on the type of formula (oil-based applications tend to work longer than water- or alcohol-based ones), the conditions, and individual chemistry (some people are just more attractive to bugs — see Don't Be a Mosquito Magnet, page 74).

Keep an on eye on how it's working. Bugs won't land on you at first, but as the potency wanes, they will begin to hover or land on your skin. That's the time to reapply, before they begin actually biting.

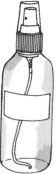

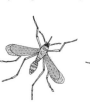

FEND-OFF OIL

This pleasantly fragranced repellent — originally published in my book *Organic Body Care Recipes* — is one of my favorites. I use it every day when bugs are at their worst. It's gentle enough to be used as bath oil, hair conditioner, scalp massage oil, after-shower oil, and all-purpose moisturizing oil. The bugs stay away, and as a bonus, my skin is very soft and conditioned. I even get occasional compliments on my unusual "perfume." If they only knew!

Note: Soybean oil is used as a base for its natural bug-repellent properties, but you can substitute your favorite lightweight base oil, such as jojoba, sunflower, almond, or grapeseed.

. . . .

15 drops each of the following essential oils:
   lemongrass, geranium, catnip
10 drops eucalyptus (species *radiata* or *globulus*) essential oil
½ cup organic soybean base oil
4-ounce spritzer, pump, or squeeze bottle

. . . .

1. Add the lemongrass, geranium, catnip, and eucalyptus essential oils to the container, then add the soybean oil. Screw the top on the bottle and shake vigorously to blend. Allow the oil to synergize for 1 hour.
2. Store at room temperature, away from heat and light; use within 1 year.

Application: Shake the bottle prior to each use. I like to put a bit of this formula onto my palms first, then massage the oil into areas that need bug protection. It is designed to penetrate quickly. If your skin feels greasy after application, you've used too much. Reapply as needed.

ESSENTIAL TICK-REPELLENT CLOTHING DROPS

This formulation combines 100 percent undiluted essential oils for a potent aroma that most humans find appealing, but ticks and flying insects absolutely abhor. When applied by the drop — to clothing, shoes, or accessories only — it creates an aromatic aura that repels these nasty pests for hours.

Caution: This is an aromatherapeutically concentrated formula, so use only by the drop as directed. Do not apply to spandex or rayon fabrics or plastic surfaces.

....

2 drops each of the following essential oils: geranium, catnip, and peppermint
1 scant tablespoon lavender essential oil
½-ounce glass bottle with screw cap

....

1. Add the geranium, catnip, peppermint, and lavender essential oils to the storage container. Screw the top on the bottle and shake vigorously to blend. Allow the oil to synergize for 1 hour.
2. Store at room temperature, away from heat and light; use within 2 years. Do not store the bottle with a dropper top, as the strong vapors will degrade the rubber tip. Store only with a screw cap.

Application: Shake well before using. Apply a few drops to your hat, bandanna or neck scarf, lower leg and hem of pants, hem of untucked shirt, cuffs or ends of shirt sleeves, inside shirt collar, and on socks. Reapply up to 3 times per day.

BUG-ME-NOT BALM

This formula has a woodsy, somewhat nutty, earthy, green herbal aroma that is generally pleasing but rather potent. Those who prefer a convenient, solid repellent will find it to their liking.

Note: I use soybean oil for its bug-repelling properties, but any lightweight base oil will do.

3 **tablespoons** organic soybean base oil

2 **teaspoons** neem base oil

2 **teaspoons** beeswax

6 **drops** each of the following essential oils: lemongrass, rosemary, cedarwood, thyme (chemotype linalool)

Small saucepan; stirring utensil; 2-ounce jar or tin

1. Warm the base oils and the beeswax over low heat until the wax is just melted. Stir the mixture gently a few times. Remove from the heat and allow the blend to cool for 5 minutes. Add the lemongrass, rosemary, cedarwood, and thyme essential oils and stir a few more times.

2. Pour into storage container(s) and cap. Allow the balm to set and synergize for 1 hour. I like to store this formula in small containers that I keep handy in my car, my purse, and my backpack, in case I need bug protection.

3. Store at room temperature, away from heat and light; use within 1 year.

Application: If wearing long pants and sleeves, dab on exposed skin, or apply a very light coating to bare arms and legs. Don't forget your temples, earlobes, the back of your neck, and the top of your head!

GERANIUM TICK-REPELLENT BALM

Geranium (rose geranium) essential oil is an amazing natural repellent and insecticide — bugs of all kinds hate it, but especially ticks. This convenient solid repellent with a fresh, rosy aroma really works to make you less attractive to ticks and flying insects. I like to store it in small containers in my car, my purse, or my backpack.
Note: Soybean oil has bug-repellent properties, but you can substitute jojoba, sunflower, grapeseed, or almond, if desired.

7 tablespoons organic soybean base oil
1–2 tablespoons beeswax (use the larger amount for a firmer balm)
48 drops geranium essential oil
Small saucepan; stirring utensil; 4-ounce jar or tin

1. Warm the base oil and the beeswax over low heat until the wax is just melted. Stir the mixture gently, then remove from the heat and allow to cool for 5 minutes. Add the geranium essential oil and stir a few more times.
2. Pour into storage container(s) and cap. Allow the balm to set and synergize for 1 hour.
3. Store at room temperature, away from heat and light; use within 1 year.

Application: If wearing long sleeves and long pants, dab a little on any entry point for biting bugs, such as wrists and ankles, as well as on temples, earlobes, nape of neck, and top of head. If wearing shorts and short sleeves, also apply a light coating to bare arms and legs. Reapply as needed.

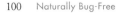

BUG-BAN BALM

One of my favorite solid insect-repellent balms, this one uses shea butter as the base. It penetrates quickly to create a pleasingly fragrant, skin-conditioning bug barrier.

....

4 tablespoons shea butter (refined or unrefined)

20 drops lavender essential oil

14 drops thyme (chemotype linalool) essential oil

14 drops geranium essential oil

Small saucepan; stirring utensil; 2-ounce jar or tin

....

1. Warm the shea butter over low heat until it has just melted. Remove from the heat and allow to cool for 5 minutes. Add the lavender, thyme, and geranium essential oils and stir a few times to blend. Pour into storage container, cap, and set aside until the balm has thickened. Unlike beeswax, shea butter can take a long time to completely thicken, and this formula may need up to 24 hours, depending on the temperature in your home. When ready, the balm will be very thick, semi-hard, and white (or creamy yellow if you use unrefined shea butter).

2. Store at room temperature, away from heat and light; use within 1 year.

Application: If wearing long sleeves and long pants, dab a little on any entry point for biting bugs, such as wrists and ankles, as well as on temples, earlobes, nape of neck, and top of head. If wearing shorts and short sleeves, also apply a light coating to bare arms and legs. Reapply as needed.

COCONUT BODY OIL #1: LIGHT, COOL FLORAL

This blend makes a silky-smooth, moisturizing body oil that just happens to fend off mildly to moderately hungry insects. Condition your skin while naturally repelling bugs — what a concept! The aroma of the essential oils is scarcely noticeable at first, but the lovely scent develops when this blend is massaged into warm skin.

....

10 drops each of the following essential oils: eucalyptus, geranium, lavender, sweet orange, and peppermint
½ cup extra-virgin, unrefined coconut base oil
4-ounce plastic squeeze bottle

....

1. Add the eucalyptus, geranium, lavender, sweet orange, and peppermint essential oils to the bottle, then add the coconut oil. If the coconut oil is solid or semi-solid, simply set the container in a shallow pan of hot water to liquefy — it melts quickly. Screw the top on the bottle and shake vigorously to blend. Allow the oil to synergize for 1 hour.

2. Store at room temperature, away from heat and light; use within 1 year.

Application: Shake the bottle prior to each use. (Coconut oil solidifies below 76°F [25°C]. If this happens, simply warm the bottle in a shallow pan of hot water or set it in a sunny window for 30 minutes or so to liquefy.) Because the oil penetrates the skin so easily, you can apply it to damp or dry skin. If your skin feels greasy after application, you've used too much. Reapply as needed to repel bugs.

COCONUT BODY OIL #2: WARM, WOODSY HERBAL

Here's another coconut oil–based body oil recipe blend that's effective against mildly to moderately hungry bugs. This one has a warmer, woodsy herbal aroma that becomes detectable after it is massaged into warm skin.

. . . .

15 drops rosemary essential oil

10 drops cedarwood essential oil

8 drops lemongrass essential oil

7 drops tea tree essential oil

4 drops lemon essential oil

4 drops patchouli essential oil

½ cup extra-virgin, unrefined coconut base oil

4-ounce plastic squeeze bottle

. . . .

1. Follow the instructions for Coconut Body Oil #1, substituting these essential oils.

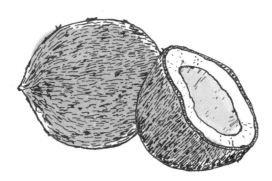

EDIBLE MOSQUITO & TICK REPELLENTS

Some readers might be skeptical about this — "Seriously, bug repellents that I can eat?" — but it's true. Eating certain foods on a regular basis makes you less attractive to blood-seeking pests. Just make sure the whole family does it, so you aren't repelling each other!

GARLIC. Mosquitoes and ticks abhor the taste of garlicky blood. Garlic is rich in a variety of powerful sulfur-containing compounds — the best known is allicin — that are responsible for its pungent odor, as well as its antiviral, antibiotic, antifungal, and vermicidal properties, among other health-promoting effects. Sulfur compounds can also be detected on your breath as well in your sweat and sebum (the natural oil on your skin), resulting in a bug-repelling aura around your body.

In order to release the potent bug-repelling compounds, garlic cloves must first be finely chopped and exposed to air. Eat them raw in salads, as a tapenade, or in garlic butter. For cooking, wait 10 minutes after chopping before adding minced garlic to a hot pan. Try to eat one to two cloves of garlic per day during bug season.

STRONG-TASTING VEGETABLES. Other yummy foods that infuse your blood with sulfur are: kale, broccoli, and cabbage; mustard, collard, and turnip greens; onions, shallots, scallions, and chives. As an extra benefit, these foods are also rich in calcium, magnesium, potassium, folic acid, and bountiful antioxidants.

B VITAMINS. Mosquitoes and ticks dislike the flavor and scent of human sweat impregnated with B vitamins, especially B_1 (thiamine). The richest food sources of thiamine include brewer's or nutritional yeast (not baking yeast), brown rice and rice bran, egg yolks, legumes, blackstrap molasses, wheat germ, peanuts, whole grains, fish, peas, organic pork, and poultry.

Adding a natural B-complex supplement that includes up to 50 mg of B_1 to your daily diet might be wise if you happen to live in an area heavily infested with mosquitoes and ticks. The B vitamins are water soluble, so any excess that you don't use nutritionally will leave your body via your sweat, breath, and urine — forming a bite-free vapor barrier between you and the bugs!

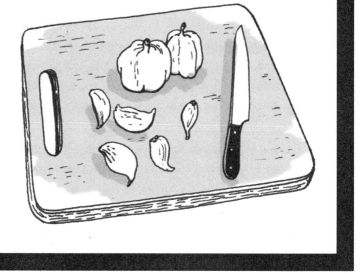

Keep Mosquitoes in Check While Dining on Your Deck

According to the American Mosquito Control Association, "Mosquitoes are relatively weak fliers, so placing a large fan on your deck can provide a low-tech solution." Another effective idea, and a more attractive one, is the addition of a chiminea or backyard brazier to your deck decor. Offering a welcoming glow and comforting warmth, they emit just enough smoke to deter biting bugs. The smoke can be aromatically enhanced by adding 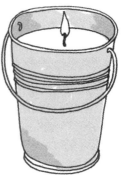 fragrant woods such as pinion, mesquite, apple, or resinous dry pine, creating a most alluring outdoor atmosphere.

And let's not forget the old standbys for creating a bug-repelling shield around your deck: burning citronella candles, tiki torches, and incense sticks or plain punks, along with moxa sticks and herbal smudge blends (see Outdoor Repellent Smudge, page 85).

Tinctures and Infusions

HERBAL REPELLENT BASE #1:
TINCTURE OF YARROW, CATNIP & PENNYROYAL

An alcohol extract of three of nature's finest insect-repelling herbs plus a little bit of insecticidal neem base oil, the basic formula has a rather strong, earthy, nutty, herby scent. Use it as is or enhance it with one of the suggested essential oil combinations, each creating a potent synergistic blend that will knock the socks off buzzing, biting bugs.

As a bonus, this formula also serves as a pretty darn good household insecticide. Spray it directly on bugs, on their nests, and on spider webs as often as necessary.

Note: The base formula requires 4 weeks to make the extract, so plan ahead. Do not spray on light-colored fabrics, wallpaper, carpeting, or unfinished wood surfaces, as it will stain.

....

½ **cup** dried or 1 cup fresh catnip leaves and flowers (a 50/50 mix is recommended; if only the leaves are available, that's fine)

½ **cup** dried or 1 cup fresh pennyroyal leaves

½ **cup** dried or 1 cup fresh yarrow leaves and flowers (a 50/50 mix is recommended; if only the leaves are available, that's fine)

1 **teaspoon** vegetable glycerin

1 **teaspoon** neem base oil

4 **cups** unflavored vodka (approximate amount)

1-quart canning jar; plastic wrap; fine-mesh strainer and fine filter; funnel; 8- or 16-ounce storage containers and spritzer bottles

1. If you're using fresh herbs, cut or tear them (including bits of stem) into smaller pieces to expose more surface area during maceration (extraction). Place the catnip, pennyroyal, and yarrow, along with the glycerin and neem oil, in a 1-quart canning jar. Pour the vodka over them to within ½ inch of the top of the jar. Place a piece of plastic wrap over the mouth of the jar (to prevent the metal lid from coming into contact with the jar's contents), then screw on the lid. Shake the mixture for about 30 seconds. After 24 hours, top up with more vodka if necessary. The herbs will settle a bit in the jar, but that's okay.

2. Store the jar in a cool, dark place for 4 weeks so that the vodka can extract the valuable chemical components from the herbs. Shake the jar for 15 to 30 seconds each day.

3. At the end of the 4 weeks, strain the herbs through a fine-mesh strainer lined with a fine filter such as muslin or, preferably, a paper coffee filter, then strain again if necessary to remove all herb debris. Press or squeeze the herbs to release all the valuable herbal extract. Discard the marc. The resulting tincture will be medium-golden brown in color. Pour the liquid into labeled storage containers.

4. Store at room temperature, away from heat and light; use within 2 years.

Application: Shake immediately before use. Spray liberally onto skin as needed — approximately every 20 to 30 minutes.

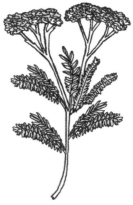

To make the following formulas: Combine the Herbal Repellent Base #1, the water, and all the essential oils in an 8-ounce glass or plastic spray bottle. Shake vigorously to blend. Allow the solution to synergize for 1 hour.

Citrus Fresh

½ **cup** Herbal Repellent Base #1

½ **cup** purified water

18 drops lemongrass essential oil

12 drops lemon eucalyptus (eucalyptus citriodora, *Corymbia citrio-dora*; or substitute *E. globulus*) essential oil

10 drops citronella essential oil

8 drops lemon essential oil

Clean & Green

½ **cup** Herbal Repellent Base #1

½ **cup** purified water

18 drops lavender essential oil

15 drops rosemary essential oil

15 drops thyme (chemotype linalool) essential oil

Mighty Mint

½ **cup** Herbal Repellent #1

½ **cup** purified water

15 drops catnip essential oil

15 drops peppermint essential oil

5 drops rosemary essential oil

HERBAL REPELLENT BASE #2: TINCTURE OF TANSY & CATNIP

Here's another of my favorite alcohol extracts, which again features catnip but with tansy and a little bit of insecticidal neem base oil added to the mix. This basic formula can be used as is (it has an earthy, nutty, green scent) or enhanced with one of the suggested essential oil combinations, each creating a potent blend that will send aggravating attackers in the opposite direction.

As a bonus, this formula serves as a wonderfully effective household insecticide, especially against ants, cockroaches, silverfish, earwigs, moths, and spiders. Simply spray directly on bugs, on their nests, and on spider webs as often as necessary.

Note: The base formula requires 4 weeks to make the extract, so plan ahead. Do not spray on light-colored fabrics, wallpaper, carpeting, or unfinished wood surfaces, as it will stain.

....

¾ **cup** dried or 1½ cups fresh catnip leaves and flowers (a 50/50 mix is recommended; if only the leaves are available, that's fine)

¾ **cup** dried or 1½ cups fresh tansy leaves and flowers (a 50/50 mix is recommended; if only the leaves are available, that's fine)

1 **teaspoon** neem base oil

1 **teaspoon** vegetable glycerin

4 **cups** unflavored vodka (approximate amount)

1-quart canning jar; plastic wrap; fine-mesh strainer and fine filter; funnel; 8- or 16-ounce storage containers and spritzer bottles

1. If you're using fresh herbs, cut or tear them (including bits of stem) into smaller pieces to expose more surface area during maceration (extraction). Place the catnip and tansy, along with the neem oil and glycerin, in a 1-quart canning jar and pour the vodka over them, so that it comes to within ½ inch of the top of the jar. Place a piece of plastic wrap over the mouth of the jar (to prevent the metal lid from coming into contact with the jar's contents), then screw on the lid. Shake the mixture for about 30 seconds. After 24 hours, top up with more vodka if necessary. The herbs will settle a bit in the jar, but that's okay.

2. Store the jar in a cool, dark place for 4 weeks so that the vodka can extract the valuable chemical components from the herbs. Shake the jar for 15 to 30 seconds each day.

3. At the end of the 4 weeks, strain the herbs through a fine-mesh strainer lined with a fine filter such as muslin or, preferably, a paper coffee filter, then strain again if necessary to remove all herb debris. Press or squeeze the herbs to release all the valuable herbal extract. Discard the marc. The resulting tincture will be a medium-golden brown in color. Pour the liquid into labeled storage containers.

4. Store at room temperature, away from heat and light; use within 2 years.

Application: Shake immediately before use. Spray liberally onto skin as needed — approximately every 20 to 30 minutes.

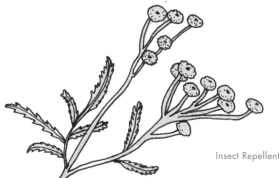

To make the following formulas: Combine the Herbal Repellent Base #2, the water, and all the essential oils in an 8-ounce glass or plastic spray bottle. Shake vigorously to blend. Allow the solution to synergize for 1 hour.

Woodsy Citrus

½ **cup** of Herbal Repellent Base #2
½ **cup** purified water
20 drops cedarwood essential oil
15 drops eucalyptus essential oil
8 drops sweet orange essential oil
5 drops citronella essential oil

Green Floral

½ **cup** of Herbal Repellent Base #2
½ **cup** purified water
18 drops lavender essential oil
15 drops rosemary essential oil
15 drops geranium essential oil

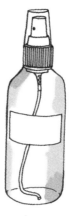

HERBAL REPELLENT BASE #3:
INFUSED OIL OF PENNYROYAL & TANSY

This recipe is an infused oil blend of two potent bug-repellent herbs. The basic formula can be used as is (it has a mild, earthy-green scent) or enhanced with one of the suggested essential oil combinations.

Note: Soybean oil is used as a base for its natural bug-repellent properties, but you can substitute your favorite lightweight, organic base oil such as jojoba, grapeseed, sunflower, or almond.

....

¾ **cup** dried or 1½ cups fresh pennyroyal leaves

¾ **cup** dried or 1½ cups fresh tansy leaves and flowers (a 50/50 mix is recommended; if only the leaves are available, that's fine)

3 cups organic soybean base oil

2,000 IU vitamin E oil (as a preservative for the infused oil)

2-quart saucepan or double boiler; stirring utensil; candy or yogurt thermometer; fine-mesh strainer and fine filter; funnel; 8- or 16-ounce storage and application containers

....

1. If you're using fresh herbs, cut or tear them (including bits of stem) into smaller pieces to expose more surface area to the oil. Combine the pennyroyal and tansy with the base oil in the saucepan and stir thoroughly to blend (it should look like a thick, leafy, yellow-green soup). Bring the mixture to just shy of a simmer, 125–135°F (52–57°C). Do not let the oil actually simmer; it will degrade the quality.

2. Allow the herbs to infuse in the oil, uncovered, over low heat for 4 hours, checking the temperature every 30 minutes and adjusting the heat accordingly. Stir the mixture at the same time, as the herb

pieces tend to settle to the bottom. If you're using a double boiler, add more water to the bottom pot as necessary.

3. After 4 hours, remove the pan from the heat and allow to cool for 15 minutes. While the oil is still warm, carefully strain it through a fine-mesh strainer lined with a fine filter such as muslin or, preferably, a paper coffee filter, then strain again if necessary to remove all debris. Squeeze the herbs to extract as much of the precious oil as possible. Discard the marc.

4. Add the vitamin E oil and stir to blend. The resulting infused oil will be a rich medium-green color, varying in depth a bit depending on the base oil. Pour the finished oil into labeled storage containers.

5. Store at room temperature, away from heat and light; use within 1 year.

Application: Shake the bottle prior to each use. I like to put a bit of this formula onto my palms first, then massage it into areas that need protection. It is designed to penetrate quickly. If your skin feels greasy after application, you've used too much. Reapply as needed.

. . . .

To make the following formulas: Combine the Herbal Repellent Base #3 and all the essential oils in an 8-ounce glass or plastic spritzer or plastic squeeze bottle. Shake vigorously to blend. Allow the solution to synergize for 1 hour.

Stimulating Blend
. . . .

1 cup Herbal Repellent Base #3
25 drops rosemary essential oil
15 drops lemongrass essential oil
8 drops eucalyptus essential oil

Woodsy Spice

....

1 cup Herbal Repellent Base #3
24 drops cedarwood essential oil
15 drops tea tree essential oil
5 drops lemongrass essential oil
2 drops cinnamon bark
  essential oil
2 drops clove essential oil

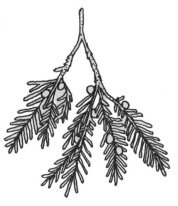

Infused Oils

An herbal infused oil has absorbed the fat-soluble properties of an herb that was soaked, or macerated, in the warmed oil for a period of time. When the maceration is complete, the herb matter (marc) is strained out and the infused oil is bottled.

Infused oils can be used on their own or blended with other infused oils to function as the main liquid ingredient when making oil-based insect-repellents for people, which include fragrant, solid balms and spray- or rub-on essential oil-blend formulations.

SUPERSENSITIVE SKIN?
TRY BUG-REPELLING ACCESSORIES

Even natural, essential oil–based repellents might irritate delicate skin, leaving the sensitive user befuddled as to what to use when venturing outdoors. The trick is to create an aromatic bug-repelling aura or "herbal haze" about your person by inoculating clothing items with pungent, powerful, insect-deterring essential oils, such as lemongrass, citronella, catnip, rosemary, eucalyptus, cedarwood, lavender, patchouli, thyme, and geranium. Try these effective tips:

- Place a drop or two of essential oil onto cotton balls and tuck them, oily side facing out, into your pants and shirt pockets and, if you wear one, your bra.

- Buy several pastel-colored bandannas and place three or four drops of essential oil on each one before venturing outside. Tie one around your neck or pin it to the back collar of your shirt; tie a couple to your belt loops and let them hang down and flap in the breeze; you can even tie a tightly rolled bandanna to each wrist.

- Add a few drops of essential oil to a pretty fabric or woven rope bracelet. It looks nice and smells good, too.

- Never forget to place a few drops of oil on the hems of pants and shorts, cuffs of shirts, and socks.

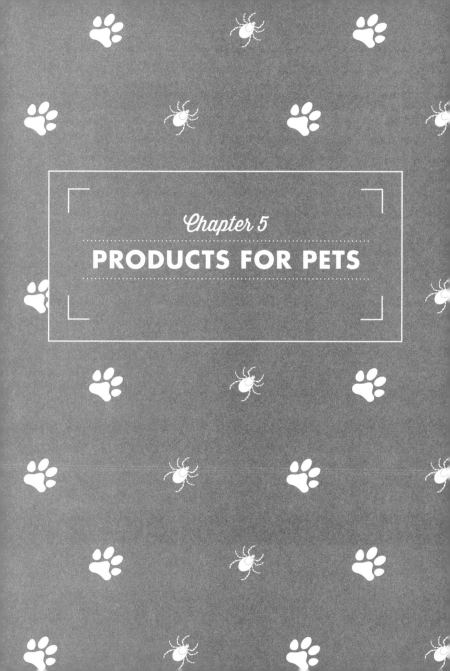

Chapter 5

PRODUCTS FOR PETS

Synthetic insecticides don't belong on the four-legged members of your family any more than they belong on your own skin. A word of caution, though: these recipes were developed for dogs and cats. I do not have experience using these recipes on any other animals, including livestock, pet rodents, or birds, so if you would like to try these or any other herb- and essential oil–based formulations on animals other than dogs or cats, please seek the advice of an herbalist and/or aromatherapist with expertise in this area, or seek out a holistic veterinarian.

Flea and Tick Biology 101

To gain some perspective on controlling these pet pests, let's first consider their life cycles — once you understand them, you can take preventive measures. Unless you have an effective, natural flea- and tick-control plan in place, which is crucial to breaking the life cycles of these parasites, ridding your pet and home of them will be next to impossible.

FLEAS

Fleas are much more than a nuisance that make pets itch and scratch. They need a warm-blooded host to provide blood as a food source and warmth for reproduction to take place. In addition to Fluffy and Fido, their "bed and breakfast" list includes wildlife, livestock, and even humans (gross!). These parasites can spread bacterial infections, induce allergic flea-bite dermatitis and sneezing, pass along tapeworms, and even cause anemia if the animal is heavily infested.

If you find even one or two fleas on your pet, an invasion is imminent, especially if it's warm and humid, conditions that they love. Here's what the life cycle of a flea looks like in your home: Adult fleas find a host — in this case your pet — feast on blood, and mate. Within a few days, the female lays tiny white eggs, which, being completely smooth, slide off your pet and sink into carpet fibers, floor cracks, pet bedding, and fabric furniture surfaces, among other areas. A flea can lay from 20 to 50 eggs at a time, for a total of about 500 to 800 during her lifetime, which averages 2 to 3 months.

The eggs hatch in a few days to 2 weeks, and the emerging larvae feed for 7 to 10 days on debris and organic matter before creating a hard-shelled cocoon and morphing into pupae. Depending on environmental conditions, the pupae develop into adult fleas anywhere from a week to a year later. The adults find a host and the cycle repeats itself — over and over and over.

A flea can lay eggs only after a blood meal. If she emerges from her cocoon and isn't able to find food, she'll die in a matter of days without reproducing. Outdoors, the cycle takes place in the soil, where adults can easily leap onto a passing host. A flea can jump about 13 inches horizontally or 7 inches vertically. In human terms, that equals about 450 or 250 feet — amazing!

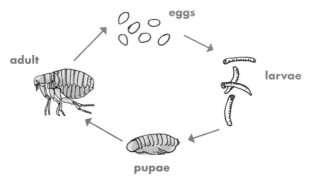

eggs

adult

larvae

pupae

FLEAS HATE GARLIC ON THEIR DOGS

Fleas feed on blood, but when they detect garlic in their food source, they will often seek another host. Depending on your dog's size, add one or two capsules of garlic extract or a few drops of garlic oil to his food a few days per week during spring, summer, and fall. Or add very small amounts of finely minced fresh garlic to their food: ⅟16 to ⅛ teaspoon for an animal under 20 pounds and up to two cloves for a very large dog (say, over 100 pounds).

Note: Garlic and other members of the Allium family can cause health problems for animals if eaten in large amounts, so don't overdo it. If your dog has digestive problems, garlic may irritate its stomach and intestines. Cats are far more sensitive to the constituents in garlic, not to mention much pickier eaters in general. Mine have always turned up their noses at it, maybe because they know it might upset their stomachs. You can also seek advice from a holistic veterinarian.

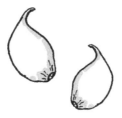

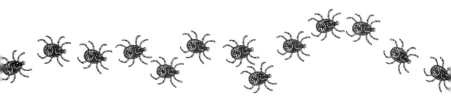

TICKS

Ticks are actually arachnids, a class of arthropods that includes scorpions, spiders, and mites. They are divided into two groups — soft bodied and hard bodied — both of which are capable of spreading disease. Ticks of every species are most active in the summer months when they're at their sexual peak. They can be found lurking in lush woods, tall grassy areas (neglected lawns and fields), and the brushy edges of your property, waiting to crawl onto any warm-blooded host who comes in close proximity.

Ticks latch on to a host, take a blood meal, then drop off and repeat the cycle until they reach adult size. This method of feeding makes them the perfect vector for transmitting disease. They lay hundreds, if not thousands, of eggs in a safe hiding place, which can include your home — horrors! The deer tick, which carries Lyme disease, takes about two years to hatch, go through its three growth stages (larva, nymph, adult) using different hosts, reproduce, and die. Other ticks go from egg to reproductive maturity in a matter of weeks.

Ticks spread several pathogens, including Rocky Mountain spotted fever, babesiosis, anaplasmosis, and Lyme disease (which tends to infect dogs much more frequently than humans and cats). Pets that live outside or often venture outdoors and are not subjected to regular grooming may attract ticks in numbers that can seriously devitalize their well-being, especially if they're small or young, leading to severe dermatitis and potentially serious anemia.

Be Proactive

Use the flea- and tick-repellent powders, sprays, and collars in this chapter, and apply the insect-control powders from chapter 6 to your hard floors, carpeting, fabric furniture, and decorative pillows, to kill fleas and ticks, including larvae. To help prevent infestations and discourage egg development, incorporate the following steps into your daily pet care and housecleaning chores, especially during peak parasite season.

COMB YOUR PETS DAILY. Even if they only venture outdoors for a few minutes, it takes just a split second for a flea or tick to hitch a ride. Adult fleas can live for many weeks, and combing removes them and any eggs. Use a special flea comb, available at pet supply stores and veterinarians' offices.

Run the comb right down to the skin, and after every two or three strokes (or as needed), remove the buildup — you'll see fur, obviously, and possibly a few (or many more) tiny brown adult fleas, plus flakes of dead skin, and teensy specks of black, dried blood (that's flea feces — yuck!). Place the debris into a jar half full of hot, soapy water. When finished, put the lid on the jar, give it a shake, and pour it down the toilet. Wash the flea comb in hot, soapy water, or douse it with rubbing alcohol or vodka and allow to dry.

SHAMPOO BOTH DOGS AND CATS. Use a flea- and tick-repelling shampoo once or twice a month to kill adult and hatchling fleas and remove any eggs. If your pet is miserably infested, shampoo once a week as an immediate comfort solution while you use other natural remedies to control the infestation in your home. See page 126 for recipes.

MAKE HERBAL BEDDING SACHETS. Place them in all the areas where your pets sleep. Your pet will smell fresh, but the fleas and ticks will not hang around. See page 132 for recipes

CHANGE PET BEDDING FREQUENTLY. At least once a week, wash blankets, zip-off bed covers, and pillow covers (and small fabric toys, if possible) in hot, soapy water. Add a few drops of geranium, rosemary, lavender, lemongrass, citronella, cedarwood, or peppermint essential oil to the wash cycle to impregnate the laundry with bug-repelling aromas.

VACUUM OFTEN. This includes not just wood floors and carpeting, but everywhere your pet sleeps or hangs out, such as sofas and chairs (don't forget under the cushions), tops of appliances, laundry baskets, rugs, closets, and so on. Add either 1 tablespoon of pure borax powder or five to ten cotton balls laced with several drops of peppermint, rosemary, eucalyptus, lemongrass, cedarwood, or geranium essential oil directly into the vacuum bag or canister prior to vacuuming. This usually kills ticks and fleas, but to be safe, dispose of vacuum bags and canister debris by sealing them tightly in a plastic bag before tossing.

MOP HARD-SURFACE FLOORS WEEKLY with the herbal repellent/disinfecting solution (see page 124). Don't forget to regularly mop concrete garage and patio floors, too, as indoor/outdoor pets often travel through these areas. This weekly procedure will help prevent other creepy-crawly bugs from taking up residence in your home, too. Bonus: your floors will be sparkling clean, and your home will smell wonderful!

Mop Solution

4 cups warm water

2 cups distilled white vinegar

½ **teaspoon** essential oil: lemon, sweet orange, thyme, rosemary, eucalyptus, lavender, cedarwood, lemongrass, or geranium

Combine in a mop bucket and use the mop to stir. Mop all surfaces, then wait until dry before walking on floors, or dry-mop the floor after washing.

INFUSE FABRIC-COVERED FURNITURE WITH ESSENTIAL OILS. Place from 1 to 3 drops of lavender, rosemary, geranium, or eucalyptus essential oil on each piece of medium- to dark-colored fabric-covered furniture (the larger the furniture, the more drops needed) every few days or so to infuse the air with parasite-repelling vapors.

Note: To avoid damaging the fabric, perform a test in an inconspicuous area first. Alternatively, to be on the safe side (or with light-colored furniture), place a drop or two of essential oil on individual cotton balls and tuck them under cushions and into zippered pillows or pillowcases.

DON'T GIVE UP!

Incorporating all of the above suggestions may seem like a lot of trouble, and you may feel like you are getting nowhere in the first week or two. Sure, it's a lot of work, but it's worth it. By consistently performing the above recommendations, you will create an aura around your home that adult fleas and ticks will find repugnant. Your home will be toxin-free (and smell refreshingly clean), your pets will be healthy and comfortable, and your sanity will remain intact.

Cat Caution

Cats are particularly sensitive to essential oils, and care must be taken to avoid any risk of toxicity. Their acute sense of smell heightens their distaste for strong odors; their thin skin allows for rapid absorption of substances into the bloodsteam; and most importantly, they lack the enzyme glucuronyl transferase, which aids in the metabolism of chemical constituents. My formulas rely primarily on herbs rather than essential oils, and any essential oils are used at extremely low rates.

Pet Shampoos

Each recipe yields about 1 cup of shampoo, which is best mixed directly in a plastic squeeze bottle. Store the container at room temperature, away from heat and light; use within 1 year.

GENERAL INSTRUCTIONS

Add the essential oils directly to the storage bottle, then add the jojoba oil, glycerin, liquid soap, and water. Screw the top on the bottle and shake gently to blend. Allow the shampoo to synergize for 1 hour. Label and date the container.

Follow the bath with the After-Shampoo Rinse for Dogs & Cats (page 129) for an added flea- and tick-repelling, aromatic boost.

FELINE FORMULA #1: GERANIUM

This nonirritating shampoo, with a trace of geranium essence, will leave your cat's fur soft and shiny.

....

2 drops geranium essential oil

½ **teaspoon** jojoba base oil

½ **teaspoon** vegetable glycerin

1 **tablespoon** liquid castile soap (lavender or almond scented); or unscented baby soap

⅞ **cup** purified water

For tips on bathing a cat, see Bathing Cats and Dogs, page 130.

FELINE FORMULA #2: CEDARWOOD

Another gentle choice, cedarwood essential oil will infuse your cat's fur with an appealing earthy-woody aroma.

....

2 drops cedarwood essential oil
½ **teaspoon** jojoba base oil
½ **teaspoon** vegetable glycerin

1 tablespoon liquid castile soap (lavender or almond scented); or unscented baby soap
⅞ **cup** purified water

For tips on bathing a cat, see Bathing Cats and Dogs, page 130.

CANINE FORMULA #1: ROSEMARY & EUCALYPTUS

Hints of rosemary and eucalyptus have excellent insect-repelling properties and aid in deodorizing a stinky coat. A definite win-win for you and your dog.

....

3 drops rosemary essential oil
3 drops eucalyptus essential oil
½ **teaspoon** jojoba base oil
½ **teaspoon** vegetable glycerin

1 tablespoon liquid castile soap, peppermint or eucalyptus scented
⅞ **cup** purified water

Application: Brush your dog thoroughly before bathing to remove loose fur and tangles. Use a tablespoon or so of shampoo for a small dog (under 20 pounds). For larger dogs, apply a quarter cup or so of shampoo, depending on the dog's size and the length of its fur.

CANINE FORMULA #2: CEDARWOOD & ORANGE

Essential oils of cedarwood and orange result in a pleasing, woodsy scent that smells great on Fido but sends bugs searching for another host.

....

3 drops cedarwood essential oil
3 drops sweet orange essential oil
½ teaspoon jojoba base oil
½ teaspoon vegetable glycerin
1 tablespoon liquid castile soap, peppermint or eucalyptus scented
⅞ cup purified water

Application: Brush your dog thoroughly before bathing to remove loose fur and tangles. For small dogs, use a tablespoon or so of shampoo. For larger dogs, apply a quarter cup or so of shampoo, depending on the dog's size and the length of its fur.

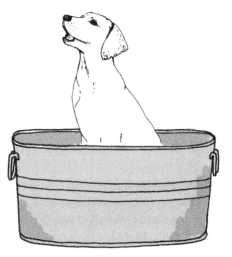

AFTER-SHAMPOO RINSE FOR DOGS & CATS

This wonderfully aromatic flea- and tick-repelling "tea" makes the perfect final rinse to use after shampooing your pet. It leaves the coat nicely conditioned and smelling ultra fresh. Prepare it a couple of hours ahead of bath time so that it can cool down before you use it.

....

½ **cup** dried or 1 cup fresh herbs (lavender buds, or the leaves of rosemary, thyme, lemon thyme, lemongrass, or eucalyptus)

2 quarts purified water

3-quart saucepan; stirring utensil; strainer and fine filter; funnel; plastic storage container, such as a gallon jug or small bucket

....

1. If using fresh herbs, first chop them up into smaller pieces or crush them using a mortar and pestle to release the potent essential oils. Bring the water to a boil and remove from heat. Add the herbs, stir gently, cover, and allow to steep for 30 minutes. Strain into the plastic storage container, cover, and allow the rinse to cool for 2 hours before using. Discard the marc or spent herbs.
2. Remaining liquid may be stored in the refrigerator for up to 3 days.

Application: Make sure the rinse is at a comfortable temperature — no need to shock your pet! After shampooing and thoroughly rinsing your pet with clear water, pour this herbal rinse over its entire body, working it into the fur. For a small to medium-size pet, 2 to 4 cups is sufficient. Use the entire amount for a medium-to-large dog. Towel off until the coat is as dry as possible.

BATHING CATS AND DOGS

Shampooing infested pets is a quick and easy way to kill fleas and wash away eggs. My mild, low-sudsing shampoos also kill bacteria resulting from flea bites, soothe skin, and leave the coat soft and clean without stripping the natural, protective oil from their skin. Dogs and especially cats are more sensitive to concentrations of essential oils than humans, so I use very small amounts in my formulations — resulting in a shampoo that is aromatically mild but still effective.

It is much easier to shampoo a dog than a cat — that's a given. Most dog owners are used to giving the occasional bath, but here are a few pointers for bathing a cat. Start by clipping their claws to reduce the chance of serious scratches. You might enlist the help of a glove-wearing assistant.

If you are blessed with a mild-mannered, trusting feline, then you may, with gentle coaxing, persuade it to tolerate a short bath in a quiet bathroom. If not, don't scare the poor thing to death by forcibly wrangling it into the water. Focus on the other weapons in your arsenal instead. Here's a general procedure that works for cats (and dogs, too), using your bathtub or a smaller container, such as a large plastic storage bin, set in the tub.

....

1. Fill the tub with a comfortable amount of lukewarm, or slightly warmer, water. Fill a couple of gallon jugs with clean, warm rinse water and set them within reach. Shake the shampoo bottle to blend the contents.

2. Set the cat in the tub (don't forget to close the door first!), keeping a firm, but gentle grip on the scruff or shoulder area. Massage the fur with water until soaked. Apply a couple of teaspoons or so of shampoo (depending on the cat's size and the length of its fur), working up a lather from the neck and down the back, including the tail, belly, and legs.

3. Wash the head last, carefully avoiding contact with the eyes, ears, and nose. You may find fleas on the face and ears as they scurry toward dry skin — just pluck them off and drown them.

4. Allow suds to remain on your pet for 3 to 5 minutes while the tub drains. Rinse the fur with clean, warm water, poured gently from the gallon jugs, until all traces of shampoo are gone.

5. Wrap your cat in towels, and dry it off as much as possible before releasing it. Don't be surprised if it flings itself around the house at first or stays away from you for a while after being treated to such an indignity!

With dogs or cats, you'll have more success if you stay calm and talk softly during the procedure. If you can avoid it, don't shampoo a sick, weak, or injured animal or one that is under 6 months old. Wait a couple of hours after your pet has eaten, and don't bathe a pet that is stressed out from visiting the vet or any other unusual event.

HERBAL PET-BEDDING SACHETS

Whether your furry friend sleeps in a blanket-filled crate or box; in a carpet-covered cat condo; or on a fleece-covered beanbag or soft pillow, tucking small bags or sachets of herbal blends in and around bedding materials is an effective way to safely deter irritating pests while keeping your pet and its sleeping area smelling fresh. Pets often have several sleeping or napping areas, so place two or more sachets in every location.

Note: Immediately after making the sachets, the essential oil fragrance (if you've added it) will be at its most potent, but it will mellow dramatically within 24 hours as it is absorbed by the herbs, so don't worry about overwhelming your dog with a lingering aroma. Cats are often quite sensitive to both the pungency and naturally occuring chemicals in essential oils, so when making sachets for feline friends, omit the essential oil.

GENERAL INSTRUCTIONS: To make the sachets, you'll need six 4- by 6-inch drawstring muslin bags or large "seal and brew" tea bags, a large bowl, and a mixing spoon.

Combine the herbs in the bowl, then add the essential oil (for dogs only), and stir again. Spoon approximately 1 cup of the mix into each bag. Label and date the bags using a permanent marker. Store leftover mixture at room temperature in an airtight container away from heat and light, and use within 1 year.

To use the sachets, place two or more bags in your pet's bedding area (the larger the pet, the more bags). Squeeze the bags every couple of days or so to release more scent. Recharge the bags by adding one drop of essential oil once per week, if desired. Replace the herbs every 2 months or so, or make new bags.

Fresh Eucalyptus

2 **cups** dried eucalyptus leaves
1 **cup** dried basil leaves
1 **cup** dried tansy leaves
  and flowers

1 **cup** dried pennyroyal leaves
1 **cup** dried peppermint leaves
15 **drops** eucalyptus essential oil
(omit for cats)

Citrus-Lavender Spice

2 **cups** dried lavender buds
1 **cup** dried cedar shavings
1 **cup** dried orange peel
1 **cup** dried lemon peel

1 **cup** dried cinnamon chips
15 **drops** cedarwood essential oil
(omit for cats)

Catnip Fair

2 **cups** dried catnip leaves and
  flowers
2 **cups** dried sage leaves
1 **cup** dried rosemary leaves

1 **cup** dried thyme leaves
15 **drops** rosemary essential oil
(omit for cats)

These blends can also be used to repel pests in kitchen and bathroom cabinets, clothing drawers, armoires, and closets. Feel free to double the essential oil amount so that the sachets have extra potency!

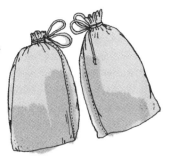

Penny's Royal Blend

2 cups dried pennyroyal leaves
2 cups dried wormwood leaves
1 cup dried thyme leaves
1 cup dried tansy leaves
and flowers

15 drops thyme essential oil,
linalool or thymol chemotype
(omit for cats)

Catnip Royale

2 cups dried catnip leaves
and flowers
2 cups dried pennyroyal leaves
2 cups dried lavender buds

10 drops peppermint essential oil
(omit if making sachets)
10 drops lavender essential oil
(omit if making sachets)

A Healthier Host Means Fewer Parasites

I can't say enough about the importance of feeding your pet
a nutrient-rich diet. That means low or no-grain kibble; real,
antibiotic- and hormone-free meat, poultry, or fish; plus essential
fats, some veggies, and other healthy foods, such as supplements
of garlic, ground pumpkin seeds, and a bit of brewer's yeast. A
pet with a super-strong immune system typically has a blood-
stream that is less attractive to fleas, ticks, and intestinal parasites,
whereas a pet that consumes an unhealthy diet might have a
compromised immune system. Check with your veterinarian
before radically changing your pet's diet.

GERANIUM TICK-REPELLENT SPRAY FOR DOGS

Several years ago while doing some research on bug-repelling essential oils, I discovered that one of my favorite oils, geranium, was recommended for using on dogs in order to keep ticks at bay. I formulated a simple water-based spray that I used to spritz on my 85-pound Irish setter before we went for our walks. It worked wonderfully well and it made his coat smell fresh, green, and slightly rosy, too! Use this spray on adult dogs over 25 pounds.

1 **scant cup** of purified water
1 **tablespoon** of plain vodka
6 **drops** of geranium essential oil
8-ounce plastic or glass spritzer bottle

1. Combine the water, vodka, and essential oil in the spritzer bottle. Cap the bottle, then shake vigorously. Shake prior to each use to recombine.

Application: Apply one spritz to your dog's hindquarters (base of tail or back of legs), one spritz along the back, and one spritz to the belly. Spritz twice onto the palm of your hand, then massage a bit onto each paw. That's it! Do not spray into your pet's face or over its entire body. Use once or twice daily and only as instructed. Store the bottle in a dark, cool place for up to 1 year.

HERBAL AURA FLEA COLLARS

Chemical-infused plastic flea and tick collars aren't a great option: they don't work very well, their poisons often irritate the skin beneath the collar, and vapors irritate the animal's delicate mucous membranes and respiratory tract. You also don't want children in contact with chemical pet collars. These essential oil–infused cloth collars, on the other hand, provide a gentle pest-repelling "halo" around your pet, pose no threat with irritating toxins, and leave their fur smelling fresh and herby. They are easy to make, completely safe as long as your pet can't lick them, and can be recharged weekly.

While an herbal collar won't give total protection against fleas and ticks, it can be a part of your arsenal against these parasites. These collars are for small adult dogs and cats under 25 pounds but are not recommended for medium-to-large animals, as the herbal aroma from the collar will not encompass or surround their bodies and reach the extremities, which is true also of chemical collars. Fleas may avoid the neck and head area only to gather elsewhere on the body.

GENERAL INSTRUCTIONS: Soft, nylon web or cotton tape collars can be found in pet supply stores and many large grocery stores. If you're feeling crafty, fashion a collar from a length of ½- or ⅜-inch wide webbing or tape and a buckle — both can be found at craft or fabric stores.

To make one collar, follow these instructions, using the ingredients listed for the particular blend. Because cats are quite sensitive to the naturally occuring chemical components in essential oils and intense aromas, I use fewer drops in their formulas, and I choose oils that are less pungent, though still effective. The garlic odor in the Savory blend may linger for a while but will fade.

1. Add the vodka and essential oils to a very small bowl, and stir to blend. Lay the collar flat on a baking sheet, and pour the mixture directly over the length of collar until fully absorbed. Air-dry until at least semidry.
2. Collars are meant to be used as soon as they have dried enough to be comfortable; do not store them. Recharge the collar weekly by soaking it in fresh formula.

Cautions: Do not use on cats or dogs under the age of 1 year, and never apply the essential oil blend directly to any pet's fur.

Cat Collar #1: Rosy Floral

1 teaspoon unflavored vodka   **1 drop** geranium essential oil

Cat Collar #2: Mild Cedar

1 teaspoon unflavored vodka   **1 drop** cedarwood essential oil

Dog Collar #1: Savory Herb

1 teaspoon unflavored vodka   **1 drop** thyme essential oil
1 drop rosemary essential oil   garlic oil from 1 small capsule

Dog Collar #2: Cedarwood-Lemongrass

1 teaspoon unflavored vodka   **1 drop** cedarwood essential oil
1 drop eucalyptus essential oil   **1 drop** lemongrass essential oil

SAGE, ROSEMARY, AND BASIL

Powdered rosemary is particularly effective against ticks, while sage makes fleas hop elsewhere. Infused basil tea used as a spray creates an effective tick-repelling herbal haze around your pet.

Herbal Powders

Grind ½ to 1 cup of dried, whole sage and/or rosemary leaves in a coffee grinder, blender, or food processor.
To use, massage the powder into the fur, all the way down to the skin. Most pets will shake off a good bit, so apply it outdoors, but enough should remain to be effective. Store powder in an airtight container by the door where you can apply it before every outing.

Notes: Powdered sage is readily available at most grocery stores, and both herbs can be found in powdered form online. Use this technique to make almost any herbal powder, including lavender, neem leaf, and lemongrass.

Basil Infusion Spray

Pour 2 cups of boiling water over 2 tablespoons of dried basil or 4 heaping tablespoons of fresh, finely chopped basil leaves. Cover, and steep for 2 hours. Strain the liquid, then pour into a 16-ounce plastic spray bottle. Store in the refrigerator for up to 7 days.

To use, spray your pet's entire body before every outing; the effect lasts several hours. If your pet spends most of its time outdoors, reapply several times per day in the height of tick season.

FLEA- & TICK-CONTROL POWDERS

These mildly aromatic recipes combine insecticidal herbs and essential oils with food-grade diatomaceous earth (DE) and bentonite clay (BC), two mineral-rich substances that deliver a double-pronged deathblow to fleas and unattached ticks. They are powerful desiccants, due to the abrasive action of the silica on the parasite's exoskeleton, and they also clog the insect's breathing channels, leading to death within 24 to 72 hours.

These powders work remarkably well when applied regularly, once or twice per week, especially during the warmer months. No worries about your pets licking themselves, either — ingesting DE and BC will even add valuable minerals to their dietary intake, and the high silica content assists as a natural dewormer. Additionally, the powder acts as a deodorizer and dry shampoo, leaving your pet's coat smelling fresh and clean.

GENERAL INSTRUCTIONS: Each of the recipes yields 2 cups of powder. You'll need a bowl and whisk, and plastic, cardboard, metal, or glass application and storage containers. A good application container is a recycled herb or spice jar with a perforated lid.

Combine the DE and/or BC with other dry ingredients specified in a medium bowl and gently whisk to blend. Add the essential oils, scattering the drops around the powder, and whisk again to combine. Loosely spoon the mixture into the container(s), then shake vigorously for about 30 seconds. Label and date the powder. Allow the powder to synergize for 24 hours prior to use. Store at room temperature, away from heat and light; use within 1 year.

Application: To ensure maximum effectiveness, sprinkle the powder evenly and uniformly from nose to tail, and as close to the skin as possible, massaging it in really well. Fleas and ticks will rush to any part of your pet that is dust-free, so address the entire face, ears, genitals, anus, and between the toes. When applying to the face, be extra careful not to get powder in the eyes, nose, or mouth, as it is irritating to mucous membranes. Repeat once or twice per week, as needed, to control fleas and ticks.

Caution: When treating mature pets under 5 pounds or young kittens and puppies, carefully apply very small amounts of powder to one section of the body at a time, massaging it into the skin very gently to minimize dust.

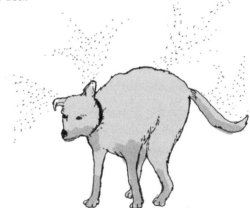

To prevent making a dust cloud in your home, I suggest powdering both your indoor and outdoor pets outside, keeping them controlled with a comfortable harness and leash (this includes cats). Most pets will shake off much of the powder immediately after being treated, but if you've massaged it close to the skin, a sufficient amount should remain to do the job.

"Shoo, Flea, Don't Bother Me" Powder

Rosemary and cedarwood give this powder a pleasant, light, woody-green scent. Be aware that the black walnut hull powder can temporarily darken blond or white fur.

....

1 cup food-grade
   diatomaceous earth
½ cup bentonite clay powder
¼ cup rosemary leaf powder

¼ cup black walnut hull powder
5 drops cedarwood essential oil
5 drops rosemary essential oil

Bite Ban Flea & Tick Powder

Lemongrass and neem, two of nature's best pest-repelling herbs, come together in this pleasant, earthy-lemony scented powder.

....

1½ cups food-grade
   diatomaceous earth
¼ cup lemongrass powder

¼ cup neem leaf powder
10 drops lemongrass essential oil

Bugs-Be-Gone Powder

I tend to favor light, floral aromas in the spring and summer, which is when I apply pest-repelling powders to my indoor cats, so this delicate lavender-rose scented formula is a favorite — it makes their fur smell oh-so-nice!

....

1 cup food-grade
   diatomaceous earth
½ cup neem leaf powder

½ cup lavender flower powder
10 drops geranium essential oil

Note: Omit essential oils in powders made for cats and for dogs under one year old.

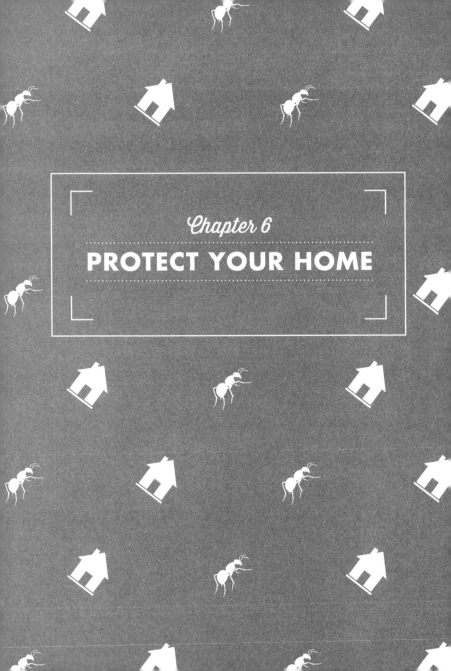

Chapter 6

PROTECT YOUR HOME

The myriad environmental and health warnings and precautions written in tiny print on the back of every synthetic insecticide are enough to scare the heck out of anyone. But fortunately you have other options, unless you have damaging infestations of termites, carpenter ants or bees, or wood-boring beetles; rodent nests in your walls; or bats in your attic — these situations need professional attention.

I've created plenty of easy-to-prepare recipes for effective herbal products that safely rid your home of insects and pests without creating toxic residues or vapors. These recipes also leave your home smelling fresh and clean — you can't say that about mothballs and chemical foggers!

While major rodent infestations warrant professional attention, this chapter does offer a few solutions to repel mice: see Hippie-Dippy Mint (page 152), Refreshing Lavender-Mint (page 152), Bugs-at-Bay (page 153), Vetiver Pest Chaser (page 154), Anti-Moth Combo (page 154), and Freeze-n-Fry Insecticide (page 164).

Prevention Is the Best Solution

Bugs have a keen sense of smell and are drawn to anything that even remotely smacks of sustenance. This can include household dirt, human and pet hair and dander, bits of litter box matter (yuck!), and, of course, any kind of food, be it crumbs or sticky smears. Many bugs are particularly drawn to sugary foods. The cleaner your home, the less attractive it will be to unwanted "guests." Here are some simple ways to keep pests at bay.

- Vacuum floors and furniture frequently.
- Shampoo or spot-treat carpets to remove food spills and pet accidents.
- Wipe up spills immediately.
- Regularly clean beneath appliances
- Keep pet-feeding areas and bowls clean. If pests are a problem, don't leave bowls out at night.
- Store pantry items in tightly sealed containers; this includes pet food and birdseed that may be stored in the garage. Put food waste in lidded garbage cans.
- Many bugs love the smell of sweat, so don't let dirty laundry pile up on floors or overflow from the laundry bin.

Bugs seek out damp, dark, crowded places. Keep the basement and garage dry, scrupulously clean, and clutter-free. Same goes for bathrooms, laundry rooms, and cabinets. Here are some other household habits and hazards to look out for.

- Stacks of old newspapers and magazines make great hiding places. So do boxes and bags of stuff you think you "might use sometime."
- Trim back or remove foundation plantings that are too close to the house and might hold moisture against the siding or roof. Keep leaves from piling up against the house, too.

- Broken window screens and drafty windows and doors give bugs easy access to your home. Rotting wood is another open invitation, so keep sills and other entry points well maintained. Store supplies of firewood and lumber under cover and away from the foundation.

- Leaky pipes attract bugs looking for a cool drink. Loose wallpaper attracts cockroaches and silverfish that find the paste appetizing.

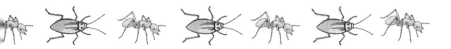

Outside Pests Coming Inside?

Mosquitoes, flies, no-see-ums, midges, and gnats can be a problem inside your home, too, not just outdoors. The most effective way to reduce a local population of mosquitoes and other moisture-loving insects around your home is to eliminate sources of standing water, such as clogged gutters, planters, birdbaths, old discarded tires, tree stump holes, unused livestock watering troughs, and abandoned fish ponds and swimming pools. Soggy compost piles also attract myriad mosquitoes, flies, and other water-seeking bugs. Make sure your compost pile has sufficient drainage, is covered with a thick layer of leaves or grass clippings, and is far away from your living quarters.

BUGS IN MY FOOD — GROSS!

Pantry moths and flour and grain beetles and mites set up camp in many kinds of bagged and packaged dry food — grains and cereals, flour and baking mixes, beans, nuts, dried fruit, bird-seed, and pet kibble — especially if such foods are past their freshness date, and where the environment is warm. Often the eggs are already in these foods when you purchase them, so you may suddenly have a problem that spreads to other packages. All you can do with infested foods is toss them and thoroughly clean out the pantry or cupboards where they were stored.

To prevent the problem from occurring, store cereal, pasta, crackers, and other products in airtight containers in a dark, cool cabinet. Some people put all flour, whole grains, and fresh nuts in the refrigerator or freezer, in tightly sealed bags or plastic containers. Keep an eye on expiration dates and rotate your pantry supplies.

Bay leaves, dried chile peppers, and whole black peppercorns are an effective deterrent sprinkled on shelves and in drawers or combined in equal proportions and put into sachet bags. Toss a few bay leaves into bags of birdseed or pet kibble before sealing them in storage tubs.

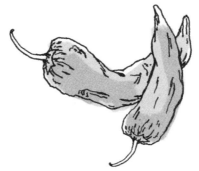

USE A DIFFUSER

An ultrasonic aromatic diffuser sprays a very fine mist of water and essential oil, sending a stream of activated ingredients into the air to deter flying pests. One relatively inexpensive machine freshens and humidifies a large room for hours.

Try these essential oils to fend off the following pests:

- All flying insects: geranium; lavender with eucalyptus OR rosemary; lemon and peppermint

- Moths: lavender, alone or with patchouli OR peppermint

- Flies: peppermint and clove

Caution: Do not use a diffuser in a room with any caged animal, particularly birds, but also rodents, reptiles, and dogs or cats in crates. The vapors may cause adverse reactions.

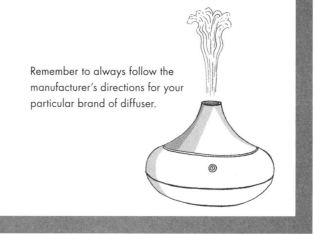

Remember to always follow the manufacturer's directions for your particular brand of diffuser.

Cleaning Sprays

Clean and disinfect your bathroom and kitchen countertops and cabinets, including both the doors and interior spaces — where insects of all kinds like to hide and make a mess — with these wonderfully aromatic, insect-repelling sprays that also aid in preventing mold and mildew. Homemade, multipurpose housekeeping products really stretch your budget — that's a good thing!

LEMON-THYME CLEANING SPRAY

If you love the clean, uplifting scent of lemons, then you'll like this formula, but the bugs won't! They especially loathe lemon essential oil.

....

1¾ **cups** purified water

¼ **cup** white vinegar

2 **teaspoons** borax

2 **teaspoons** liquid castile soap, unscented, or peppermint or eucalyptus scented

15 **drops** lemon essential oil

5 **drops** thyme essential oil, linalool or thymol chemotype

Funnel; 16-ounce spritzer bottle

....

1. Add the water, vinegar, and borax to the bottle. Screw the top on the bottle and shake vigorously until the borax is nearly dissolved, which may take a minute or two; then add the liquid soap and essential oils of lemon and thyme. Cap the bottle, and

this time shake very gently for about a minute. Allow the spray to synergize for 1 hour. **Note:** You must make this formula exactly as directed; otherwise the soap may not stay in solution and will instead transform into little waxy blobs.

2. Store at room temperature, away from heat and light; use within 1 year.

Application: Shake gently before each use. Spray generously on countertop and cabinet surfaces and wipe with a damp cloth or sponge. Follow with a dry cloth or towel.

ROSEMARY-MINT CLEANING SPRAY

The stimulating blend of rosemary and peppermint essential oils, two plant extracts that are especially unappealing to bugs, will leave your home smelling clean and welcoming to everyone, that is, except pests!

....

1¾ **cups** purified water

¼ **cup** white vinegar

2 teaspoons borax

2 teaspoons liquid castile soap, peppermint or eucalyptus scented

10 drops peppermint essential oil

10 drops rosemary essential oil

16-ounce spritzer bottle

Follow the instructions for Lemon-Thyme Cleaning Spray, substituting these essential oils.

Got Centipedes in Your Basement?

These many-legged beneficial insects actually prey on the cockroaches, flies, and moths that live in your home, especially in cool basements. So if you find a centipede or two, it indicates that other bugs are about. Time for some good herbal housecleaning!

Bug-Free Potpourris

Try an old-fashioned way of ridding your living quarters of clothing and pantry moths, ants, spiders, flour and grain beetles, silverfish, earwigs, and cockroaches and their ilk by utilizing one of the easiest pest repellents you can make: herbal potpourri. Homeowners have been using blends of pungent herbs for centuries to prevent crawling and flying vermin from setting up shop. They're inexpensive, effective, nontoxic, and "scent-sational"! No matter what's bugging you, there's an herb or potpourri blend to suit your pest-controlling needs.

BASIC POTPOURRI DIRECTIONS

These simple steps apply to the eight recipe blends that follow —
each recipe yields approximately 3 cups of potpourri.

1. Combine all the ingredients in a widemouthed, quart-size glass jar
   (a canning jar works well), and stir with a spoon or chopstick until
   well blended.
2. Cap the jar and leave it in a dark, cool cabinet for 72 hours so that
   the herbs can completely absorb the essential oils and the scent can
   fully develop. Give the jar a few good shakes each day.
3. To use, simply fill small decorative bowls, common custard cups,
   small muslin sachet bags, or seal-and-brew tea bags with your
   chosen blend and place them in food pantries; under beds and
   bathroom sinks; in clothing closets, drawers, and armoires; on
   open-closet clothing hangers and in garment pockets; on the kitchen
   counter; in the attic; in the basement; on the foundation sill; near
   open windows or directly on window sills; in the garage or garden
   shed; by the garbage pail; or close to heating and cooling vents.
4. Recharge the containers every couple of weeks by adding another
   drop or two of the essential oils. Just drop it in and give the bowl a
   stir or the bag a squeeze.
5. Make a new batch of potpourri every three months to maintain
   maximum bug-repelling effectiveness. Sprinkle the spent herb blend
   (which still has mild pest-deterring properties) around the edges of
   your landscaping beds or veggie garden; otherwise dump it into the
   compost pile, fireplace, or woodstove.

Hippie-Dippy Mint
Repels all flying and crawling pests, including mice.

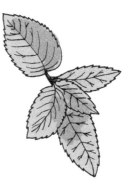

....

1 **cup** dried patchouli leaves
1 **cup** dried peppermint leaves
1 **cup** dried pennyroyal leaves
10 **drops** peppermint essential oil
10 **drops** patchouli essential oil

Refreshing Lavender-Mint
Particularly effective against ants, clothing and pantry moths, flour and grain beetles and mites, houseflies, fruit flies, gnats, mosquitoes, and mice.

....

1½ **cups** dried peppermint leaves
1 **cup** dried lavender buds
½ **cup** dried lemon peel

10 **drops** peppermint essential oil
15 **drops** lavender essential oil

Moths-Be-Gone
Best for clothing and pantry moths, but also effective against flour and grain beetles and mites, houseflies, gnats, fruit flies, mosquitoes, fleas, and ticks.

....

2 **cups** dried lavender buds
½ **cup** dried mugwort leaves
¼ **cup** dried orange peel

¼ **cup** black peppercorns
10 **drops** lavender essential oil
10 **drops** lemongrass essential oil

Bugs-at-Bay

Best for clothing and pantry moths, and flour and grain beetles and mites, but also effective against all manner of flying, crawling pests, including mice.

....

½ **cup** dried bay leaves
½ **cup** dried peppermint leaves
½ **cup** dried rosemary leaves
½ **cup** dried wormwood leaves
½ **cup** dried patchouli leaves

½ **cup** dried hot pepper flakes
3 whole nutmegs
10 drops patchouli essential oil
15 drops lemon essential oil

Classic Citrus-Cedar-Spice

Best for clothing and pantry moths, and flour and grain beetles and mites, but also effective against most creeping insects, such as cockroaches, silverfish, spiders, earwigs, pill bugs, fleas, ticks, and centipedes.

....

½ **cup** cedar shavings
½ **cup** dried rosemary leaves
½ **cup** dried lavender buds
½ **cup** dried lemon peel
½ **cup** dried orange peel
¼ **cup** cinnamon chips

¼ **cup** whole cloves
2 tablespoons black peppercorns
10 drops cinnamon bark
  essential oil
10 drops clove essential oil

Fly-Away Blend

Best for houseflies, fruit flies, gnats, mosquitoes, ants, fleas, and cockroaches, but also effective at repelling all manner of crawling insects.

1 cup dried basil leaves
½ cup dried rosemary leaves
½ cup dried eucalyptus leaves
½ cup dried tansy leaves
  and flowers
½ cup cinnamon chips
15 drops eucalyptus essential oil
10 drops rosemary essential oil

Vetiver Pest Chaser

Best for clothing and pantry moths, silverfish, ants, cockroaches, and spiders, but also works at repelling other household pests, including mice.

1 cup dried patchouli leaves
1 cup dried peppermint leaves
1 cup dried lemongrass leaves
10 drops vetiver essential oil
10 drops lemongrass essential oil

Anti-Moth Combo

Best for clothing and pantry moths, flour and grain beetles and mites, spiders, ants, and mice, but also works well at repelling most other flying and crawling household pests.

1 cup cedar shavings
1 cup dried peppermint leaves
1 cup dried pennyroyal leaves
2 tablespoons menthol crystals
20 drops camphor essential oil
20 drops cedarwood essential oil

Protect Precious Books with Vetiver

Are you an avid reader with scads of books lining shelves in your home, or perhaps have a tidy collection of antique books? Cockroaches and silverfish find the glue used in the bindings to be quite tasty (same goes for wallpaper paste). To deter these insects from destroying your most valued possessions, either apply a drop or two of vetiver essential oil to each book's binding or scatter cotton balls inoculated with the oil among your shelves. If you can find the chopped, dried root, it can be mixed with whole cloves and black peppercorns and placed in tiny bowls or sachet bags on bookshelves.

Insect-Control Powders

Sometimes a dry insecticidal powder is a better choice for eradicating bugs than a wet spray formulation, especially if you have troublesome infestations, such as fleas and ticks in your carpets or on your fabric furniture, or perhaps need to treat large areas or an entire house. My blends kill the bugs while leaving the treated area smelling fresh and clean; when applied to carpets and fabric furniture, they also deodorize fibers.

BASIC POWDER DIRECTIONS

These simple steps apply to the four recipe blends that follow. Each recipe yields about 3 cups of powder, which will treat approximately 350 square feet. Store unused amounts in an airtight container in a dark, cool, dry place, and use within 1 year.

1. Combine all the ingredients in a widemouthed, quart-size glass jar (a canning jar works well), and stir with a spoon or chopstick until well blended.
2. Cap the jar, and leave it in a dark, cool cabinet for 72 hours to ensure that the essential oil has been completely absorbed by the powders and all the scents have mingled. Give the jar a few good shakes each day.
3. To turn your jar into a shaker container, make about 12 holes in the lid with a thick nail and a hammer. To keep the air out and the powder in when processing the recipe or storing the finished product, place a small piece of plastic wrap on top of the jar, then screw on the lid. Simply remove the plastic when you want to shake out the powder.
4. To use, hold the shaker container 2 inches or less above the surface to be treated to avoid creating a cloud of dust (wearing a mask and goggles is suggested if you have respiratory allergies or sensitivities). Sprinkle ever so lightly — just enough to dust the surface. Wait 24 hours, then vacuum thoroughly. Clean the vacuum filter after each treatment, as the fine particulate matter tends to clog it. Re-treat the area once per week for three more weeks, just to ensure that any pests that are currently in egg stage are killed once they hatch.

For maximum effectiveness upon application, sprinkle the powder evenly and uniformly on all surfaces, or the crawling insects will gather on untreated areas. Dusting directly on the insects in places where they congregate or nest, or placing a powder blend unavoidably in their path is a surefire way to control traffic and potential infestations.

Bug-Bustin' Rosemary Powder

I often use this aromatically refreshing blend during the summer to prevent flea infestations in my carpeting. Rosemary powder is available from online herbal products providers, or you can make your own (see Sage, Rosemary, and Basil, page 138).

Caution: This blend contains borax — a respiratory, digestive, and mucous membrane irritant — so it is imperative that you close off treated areas to people and pets until thoroughly vacuumed.

....

1½ **cups** food-grade diatomaceous earth
¾ **cup** borax
½ **cup** rosemary leaf powder
¼ **cup** baking soda

30 **drops** peppermint or rosemary essential oil (optional, but adds a wonderful, fresh scent and enhances the insect-repelling properties)

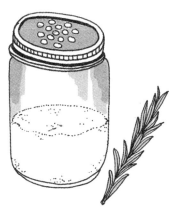

Triple-Threat Citrus Dust

The oh-so-fresh, sensory stimulating essential oils of lemon, sweet orange, and grapefruit contain limonene, a rather potent natural insecticide. When combined with diatomaceous earth, the result is a citrus-infused insect control powder that is tough on bugs, yet gentle on people and pets!

. . . .

2½ cups food-grade diatomaceous earth

½ cup baking soda

10 drops each of the following essential oils: lemon, sweet orange, and grapefruit

Flower Power Pest-Away Powder

Sprinkle this geranium-and-lavender-scented powder on your carpets, and enjoy the tranquilizing floral aroma. When I use it, my cats roll in treated areas, giving their fur the subtle aroma of a spring flower garden — not something you can say about commercial insecticide products! Lavender flower powder is available from online herbal products providers, or you can make your own (see Sage, Rosemary, and Basil, page 138).

. . . .

2½ cups food-grade diatomaceous earth

½ cup lavender flower powder

15 drops geranium essential oil

15 drops lavender essential oil

Kitchen & Bathroom Insecticidal Powder

I don't use this powder to treat large areas of my home, but simply to control kitchen and bathroom insects by sprinkling a small amount in corners and crevices whenever I see evidence of bugs setting up shop. The pepper alone acts as a strong repellent, so the bugs may just avoid your kitchen and bathroom altogether when they get an irritating whiff!

Caution: This blend contains borax — a respiratory, digestive, and mucous membrane irritant — so it is imperative that you keep children and pets away from treated areas until thoroughly vacuumed.

....

2½ cups borax
½ cup ground black pepper
40 drops eucalyptus (species *globulus*, or *Eucalyptus citriodora*) essential oil

....

Mix the borax, black pepper, and essential oil in a medium bowl.

Application: Sprinkle ½ teaspoon or so of the powder in corners of cupboards, under appliances, or wherever insects are in evidence. Leave the powder in place for about a month, then remove it by vacuuming, followed by wiping the area clean with a damp sponge inoculated with a couple of drops of peppermint, patchouli, rosemary, or eucalyptus essential oil. Re-treat if bugs make a repeat appearance.

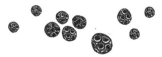

Anti-Bug Brews

My anti-bug brews are extremely simple-to-make insecticidal sprays concocted from herbal tea, essential oils, hot pepper, and liquid castile soap. They'll banish the bugs from your home while leaving a pleasing herbal scent, which additionally helps to deter future creepy-crawlers from taking up residence. Every formulation contains essential oils with potent antibacterial properties, so your home is further protected against microscopic health saboteurs.

TANSY TEA INSECTICIDAL SPRAY

Tansy, with its extremely bitter taste, contains a variety of powerful constituents, including camphor, pyrethrins, and thujone, that are toxic to a bug's central nervous system. When made into a strong infusion with essential oils of eucalyptus and lemon, plus a smidge of cayenne pepper, the result is a potent bug-bustin' brew that smells fresh to you but downright repulsive to all flying and crawling insects.

Cautions: Cayenne pepper is a strong skin irritant. Do not rub eyes or nose or put fingers in your mouth while working with it, and wash hands immediately after using. Do not spray on carpeting or fabric furniture, as this formula will stain.

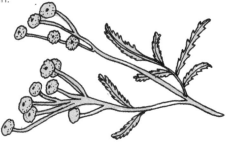

4 tablespoons fresh or 2 tablespoons dried tansy flowers and leaves

2 cups purified water

½ **teaspoon** cayenne pepper or 1 teaspoon hot pepper sauce, such as Tabasco

1 tablespoon unflavored vodka

2 teaspoons liquid castile soap, peppermint or eucalyptus scented

20 drops eucalyptus essential oil

20 drops lemon essential oil

Medium saucepan; stirring utensil; strainer and fine filter; medium bowl; funnel; 16-ounce spray bottle

···

1. If using fresh herbs, chop the herbs into small pieces or crush them with a mortar and pestle to release the potent oils. Bring the water to boil in a medium saucepan, and remove from the heat. Add the tansy and cayenne pepper or hot sauce, gently stir, cover, and allow to steep for 2 hours. Strain into a medium bowl, then pour into a storage container. Add the vodka, liquid soap, and essential oils. Screw on the top, shake vigorously to blend, and allow the spray to synergize for 1 hour.

2. Store the bottle in the refrigerator. Discard after 7 days, then make a new batch.

Application: Shake gently prior to each use. Spray the solution directly on bugs you wish to kill or in areas where you see evidence of infestation. Don't forget to spray thoroughly into insect hiding places such as cracks and crevices; around baseboards and windows and door frames; underneath and behind refrigerators, stoves, cabinets, and garbage cans; around plumbing; under sinks; in basements and attics; and in dark corners anywhere.

CITRUS "CREEPY-CRAWLY" SOLUTION

Citrus peel contains high levels of limonene, a chemical constituent with potent insecticidal properties that is also a registered active ingredient in many commercial insecticides and repellents. I make this formula often, as I love the uplifting, citrusy aroma that wafts about my house after I spray for bugs. Can't say that about Raid, now can you? This formula works for all flying and crawling insects.

Cautions: Cayenne pepper is a strong skin irritant. Do not rub eyes or nose or put fingers in your mouth while working with it, and wash hands immediately after using. Do not spray on carpeting or fabric furniture, as this formula will stain.

. . . .

20 drops lemon essential oil
20 drops orange essential oil
1 tablespoon unflavored vodka
2 teaspoons liquid castile soap, peppermint or eucalyptus scented

½ teaspoon cayenne pepper or 1 teaspoon hot pepper sauce, such as Tabasco
2 cups purified water
16-ounce spritzer bottle

. . . .

1. Add the lemon and orange essential oils directly to the storage bottle. Next, add the vodka, liquid soap, and cayenne or hot sauce, then pour in the water. Screw the top on the bottle and shake vigorously to blend. Allow the solution to synergize for 1 hour.

2. Store at room temperature, away from heat and light; use within 1 year.

Application: Shake gently prior to each use. Spray the solution directly on bugs you wish to kill or in areas where you see evidence of infestation. Don't forget to spray thoroughly into insect hiding places such as cracks and crevices; around baseboards and windows and door frames; underneath and behind refrigerators, stoves, cabinets, and garbage cans; around plumbing; under sinks; in basements and attics; and in dark corners anywhere.

EUCALYPTUS BUG ERADICATOR

Eucalyptus essential oil is capable of killing numerous soft-bodied insects or at least repelling them. I like using this spray in the winter, as the clean, fresh, stimulating scent reminds me of Vicks VapoRub. This formula works best against mosquitoes, gnats, houseflies, cockroaches, silverfish, fleas, and ticks, but it is also effective against most other flying and crawling insects.

Cautions: Cayenne pepper is a strong skin irritant. Do not rub eyes or nose or put fingers in your mouth while working with it, and wash hands immediately after using. Do not spray on carpeting or fabric furniture, as this formula will stain.

....

40 drops eucalyptus essential oil
1 tablespoon unflavored vodka
2 teaspoons liquid castile soap, peppermint or eucalyptus scented

½ teaspoon cayenne pepper or 1 teaspoon hot pepper sauce, such as Tabasco
2 cups purified water
16-ounce spritzer bottle

1. Add the eucalyptus essential oil directly to the storage bottle. Next, add the vodka, liquid soap, and cayenne or hot sauce, then pour in the water. Screw the top on the bottle and shake vigorously to blend. Allow the solution to synergize for 1 hour.
2. Store at room temperature, away from heat and light; use within 1 year.

Application: Shake gently prior to each use. Spray the solution directly on bugs you wish to kill or in areas where you see evidence of infestation. Don't forget to spray thoroughly into insect hiding places such as cracks and crevices; around baseboards and windows and door frames; underneath and behind refrigerators, stoves, cabinets, and garbage cans; around plumbing; under sinks; in basements and attics; and in dark corners anywhere.

FREEZE-N-FRY INSECTICIDE

The ultracooling menthol crystals act to chill and shock the pest's respiratory system, while at the same time the cayenne pepper burns. Sounds horrible, but this product works wonderfully well, sans toxic chemicals. After a few spritzes around the house, the strong, penetrating, mentally energizing, minty aroma will linger, which is a very good thing! This formula works for all flying and crawling insects and also deters mice.

Cautions: Cayenne pepper and menthol crystals are strong skin irritants. Do not rub eyes or nose or put fingers in your mouth while working with them, and wash hands immediately after using this formula. Do not spray on carpeting or fabric furniture, as this formula will stain.

1 tablespoon menthol crystals

1 teaspoon cayenne pepper or 2 teaspoons hot pepper sauce, such as Tabasco

1 tablespoon liquid castile soap, peppermint or eucalyptus scented

1⅞ cups unflavored vodka

16-ounce spritzer bottle

....

1. Add the menthol crystals, cayenne or hot sauce, and liquid soap to the container, then pour in the vodka. Screw the top on the bottle and shake vigorously to blend. Allow the solution to synergize for 1 hour.

Note: The menthol crystals will take approximately 20 minutes to dissolve in the alcohol. The more you shake, the more quickly they break down. If they do not break down completely, that's okay; they will still lend their strong, minty essence to the repellent.

2. Store at room temperature, away from heat and light; use within 1 year.

Application: Shake gently prior to each use. Spray the solution directly on bugs you wish to kill or in areas where you see evidence of infestation, including areas where you see mouse droppings. Don't forget to spray thoroughly into insect hiding places, such as cracks and crevices; around baseboards and windows and door frames; underneath and behind refrigerators, stoves, cabinets, and garbage cans; around plumbing; under sinks; in basements and attics; and in dark corners anywhere.

NEEM KNOCK-OUT INSECTICIDAL SPRAY

Neem oil is very effective against many bugs, and a strong antifungal as well. It has a rather pungent odor, so I've added bright, sharp rosemary and lemon essential oils. This formula works for all flying and crawling insects.

Cautions: Cayenne pepper is a strong skin irritant. Do not touch your face while working with it and wash hands immediately. This formula will stain fabric.

....

20 drops rosemary essential oil
20 drops lemon essential oil
1 tablespoon neem base oil
2 tablespoons unflavored vodka
2 teaspoons liquid castile soap, peppermint or eucalyptus scented

½ **teaspoon** cayenne pepper or 1 teaspoon hot pepper sauce, such as Tabasco
1¾ **cups** purified water
16-ounce spritzer bottle

....

1. Add the rosemary and lemon essential oils directly to the bottle. Add the neem oil, vodka, liquid soap, and cayenne or hot sauce, then pour in the water. Screw on the top and shake vigorously to blend. Allow the solution to synergize for 1 hour.
2. Store away from heat and light; use within 1 year.

Application: Shake gently prior to using. Spray directly on bugs and around infested areas, including baseboards, entry points, appliances, and plumbing.

BUG-ZAPPER BREW

This stimulating formulation can remedy just about any bug problem. It works best against spiders, silverfish, stinkbugs, cockroaches, earwigs, and ants but also for many other insects.
Caution: Will stain light-colored carpeting or fabric furniture.

....

32 drops sweet orange essential oil
12 drops patchouli essential oil
10 drops cinnamon bark essential oil
10 drops lemongrass essential oil
10 drops peppermint essential oil

6 drops tea tree essential oil
1 tablespoon unflavored vodka
2 teaspoons liquid castile soap, peppermint or eucalyptus scented
2 cups purified water
16-ounce spritzer bottle

....

1. Add the orange, patchouli, cinnamon, lemongrass, peppermint, and tea tree essential oils directly to the bottle, then pour in the vodka, liquid soap, and water. Screw on the top and shake vigorously to blend. Allow the solution to synergize for 1 hour.
2. Store away from heat and light; use within 1 year.

Application: Shake gently prior to using. Spray directly on bugs and around infested areas, including baseboards, entry points, appliances, and plumbing.

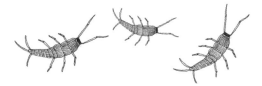

OF MICE AND MINT —
MY PERSONAL ADVENTURE

I live in a very old house — circa 1800 — complete with the original stacked granite block foundation and dirt basement floor. When I bought this quaint though rather ramshackle abode in 2006, I soon realized that late evenings were filled with the sounds of dozens of seemingly giant rodents scurrying invisibly through the ceilings and walls on both floors! My two cats had a field day (or night, I should say) galloping through the house whenever I was trying, without much success, to gain some precious shut-eye. Ever on the hunt, they rarely caught anything except the unfortunate mouse or mole that got trapped in the kitchen or bathroom.

Upon close inspection of the foundation, I discovered scads of narrow "vermin tunnels" leading through the rotten foundation sill or cracks in the granite walls, right into my basement, giving the pesky critters access into the walls, where I could hear — and sometimes even smell — them nesting. Something had to be done — and soon! I had no intention of running a boardinghouse for mice and their relatives.

Knowing that rodents are not fond of peppermint, I began to place mint strategically around my home to drive them away (I also set out lots of mousetraps baited with peanut butter). I put fresh mint sprigs and muslin-filled bags of dried mint inoculated with drops of peppermint essential oil along the foundation sill; tucked some into cracks in the foundation wall; scattered bags along with cotton balls soaked with peppermint essential oil in the attic; sprinkled dried mint as well as superstrong menthol crystals on the basement floor; and poured dried mint mixed with cayenne pepper powder into the tunnels. I also made a very potent mix of 1 teaspoon of essential oil, 1½ cups of water, and ½ cup of vodka, which I sprayed along the baseboards and around exit doors throughout the house and used to clean the windowsills.

I planted a peppermint patch in my garden so I'd always have a fresh supply. My living quarters were saturated with the superfresh essence of peppermint, and the critter problem greatly diminished, though it didn't totally disappear — it was still an old house that had been home to all kinds of crawling things for 200 years.

When the "old girl" was completely remodeled in 2012, however, the mouse, mole, bat, snake, and chipmunk problem (yeah, I encountered all of them inside the house) pretty much became a thing of the past. Occasionally, I discover a tiny furry visitor in my basement — the old stone foundation still allows one or two determined critters to get through — so peppermint has become, and will always be, my herbal ally in the continuing fight against the invaders.

Resources

The following are my tried and true favorite companies, purveyors of everything you'll need to make the recipes in this book.

Raw Materials, Packaging, Natural Health, and Personal Care Products

AromaTherapeutix
800-308-6284
www.aromatherapeutix.com

Essential oils; muslin sachet bags and storage containers; pest repellent herb blends; herbal body and health care products; and more

Aura Cacia Frontier Co-op
800-437-3301
www.auracacia.com

Essential oils, base oils, and natural skin and body care products

Bulk Herb Store
877-278-4257
www.bulkherbstore.com

Dried herbs; diatomaceous earth; teas and accessories; beeswax, bee supplements, and honey; salt; packaging supplies; books and videos

Cape Bottle Company
888-833-6307
www.capebottle.com

Wide variety of glass, plastic, and tin packaging

Eden Botanicals
855-333-6645
www.edenbotanicals.com
....

Bulk wholesale essential oils, CO_2 extracts, and absolutes for aromatherapy, natural perfumery, body and facial care

Frontier Natural Products Co-op
800-669-3275
www.frontiercoop.com
....

Essential oils and base oils; natural and organic herbs and spices; cosmetic clays; beeswax; natural skin, hair, and body care products

HOMS
888-270-5721
www.homs.com
....

Natural pesticide products for farm, home, garden, people, and pets

Jean's Greens
518-479-0471
www.jeansgreens.com
....

Health and personal care herb products; teas; herbs; essential oils and base oils; beeswax and butters; clays; packaging supplies; books

The Jojoba Company
800-256-5622
www.jojobacompany.com
....

Certified organic, unrefined, superior-quality jojoba oil

Liberty Natural Products
800-289-8427
www.libertynatural.com
....

Botanical ingredients for health and personal care; packaging supplies

Mountain Rose Herbs
800-879-3337
www.mountainroseherbs.com

Essential and base oils; hydrosols; raw ingredients; herbal health aids; pet care products; skin, hair, and body care products; packaging supplies

NYR Organic

Stephanie Tourles Independent Consultant
https://us.nyrorganic.com/shop/herbs/area/about-me/

Source of my favorite ultrasonic essential oil diffuser; luxurious, organic skin and body care; herbal remedies and aromatherapy products

Simplers Botanicals
800-229-2512
www.shopsimplers.com

Therapeutic-grade essential oils derived from ethically wildcrafted or organically grown plants; natural first-aid oils; hydrosols; infused herbal oils; herbal extracts

Specialty Bottle
206-382-1100
www.specialtybottle.com

A wide variety of glass, plastic, and tin packaging

Starwest Botanicals
800-800-4372
www.starwest-botanicals.com

Essential oils, bulk herbs and spices, herb capsules, herbal extracts, natural body care, storage containers

Index

OTHER STOREY BOOKS BY STEPHANIE L. TOURLES

. . . .

365 Ways to Energize Mind, Body & Soul
Live life to the fullest with this idea-a-day book that's filled with natural ways to stay alert and upbeat — with energizing tips and techniques including diet, exercise, health rituals, visualization, and more.

Hands-On Healing Remedies
Fill your medicine cabinet with your own all-natural, topical, handmade herbal remedies. With over 100 recipes, make linaments, balms, and essential oil blends to treat a range of health care needs such as headaches, anxiety, insomnia, cuts and scrapes, and much more.

Organic Body Care Recipes
Maintain radiantly healthy and beautiful skin, hair, and body with these fun and simple recipes for creams, scrubs, toners, and more. This wide range of beauty formulas will show you how to treat your body from head to toe with nourishing, natural ingredients.

Raw Energy
Supercharge your body with more than 100 recipes for delicious raw snacks: unprocessed, uncooked, simple, and pure. Use raw fruits, vegetables, nuts, seeds, and oils to make smoothies, trail mixes, energy bars, candies, and much more.

Raw Energy in a Glass
Enjoy more than 120 super-nutritious, super-delicious recipes for smoothies, vegan shakes, power shots, mocktails, and more, all designed to boost your health and energy using just a standard blender.

. . . .

These and other books from Storey Publishing are available wherever quality books are sold or by calling 1-800-441-5700. Visit us at *www.storey.com* or sign up for our newsletter at *www.storey.com/signup*.

31901057068779